SAVING MELISSA

7 Cs to Cure the Mental Health System

MICHAEL MACKNIAK, JD

Conservative Care, Inc.

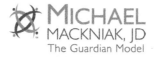

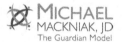

MICHAEL
MACKNIAK, JD
The Guardian Model

Michael Mackniak, JD, 750 Straits Tpke Unit 2c, Middlebury CT 06762
MichaelMackniak.com
Printed in the United States of America
First Edition
ISBN – 978-0-9974214-0-8
Library of Congress Control Number: 2016909831

DEDICATION

I dedicate *Saving Melissa* to people with mental illnesses, their families, and loved ones. I commend you all for your courage, your drive, and your fight every day. You form the backbone of this book.

With deep gratitude for allowing me to tell your story, I also dedicate this book to Robin and Melissa.

– Michael Mackniak, JD

"When we continuously improve, the next thing we do will always be the best thing we've ever done."

— Unknown

CONTENTS

FOREWORD

It was a rainy day in Waterbury, Connecticut. The building where we met back in 2001 had large letters that spelled "Broadcast Building." It once housed a studio that had long since moved away—not the place you'd go unless you had a purpose. Instead, it was where the Waterbury Mental Health Authority was renting space. I'd come to hear about a curious idea.

You would have been interested in this idea, too, if you'd have seen what I have. Since time began—and certainly since the 1960s and deinstitutionalization—our society has seen the disenfranchisement of severely mentally ill people forced from long-term care settings into the community at large. They are people whose lives are often held together by a tenuous thread. They are now expected to tolerate the complexities of life in the "real world." Basically, they are told they should be satisfied with the government aid they receive—to "just be quiet and take your medication."

But how can they maintain any semblance of normalcy in the face of an illness they sincerely believe they don't have? How can they be asked to take medication they don't believe they need? How do they tolerate medicine that makes them feel sapped of their energy, increases their appetites to the point of morbid obesity, and makes them susceptible to physical illnesses like diabetes?

What happens when they are victimized in the only neighborhoods they're able to afford? What happens when they become addicted to street drugs found in those impoverished neighborhoods? What happens when they feel they have no way out except through suicide?

This problem is faced by all of us in the field of mental health, and we struggle for solutions. On this rainy spring day in Waterbury, I was about to hear from an attorney who had an idea—a possible solution.

This attorney, Michael Mackniak, outlined a plan that had come to him through serving as a conservator to people with severe mental illness. He knew well the problems mental health professionals constantly faced. He faced them, too.

However, Attorney Mackniak was willing to ask tough questions that those of us in the industry failed to ask ourselves. He could point out what many were thinking but unable to articulate—that many severely mentally ill persons *can* live independently, work independently, and lead productive lives *with help*.

Michael's plan for help wasn't conceptual; it was proven. Having put it into action as a conservator, he had a track record of success.

In the book you are about to read, Attorney Mackniak will explain this plan to you. You will hear the personal stories that compelled him toward providing a new lifeline for the mentally ill. You will learn about the complexities of the population he serves and the challenges they confront. And you will see how the plan he offers has been a solution for many individuals, family members, loved ones, and care providers.

As you read these pages, I hope you recognize how these solutions can be part of the lives of those *you* care for, too. If you do incorporate them as I did, you can bring long-overdue solutions to people who have long deserved it.

— Dr. Paul T. Amble, MD

Chief Forensic Psychiatrist, Connecticut Department of Mental Health and Addiction Services

Assistant Clinical Professor, Yale Medical, Department of Psychiatry

INTRODUCTION

Social work has been practiced in this country since the 1960s, and theories have been developed and dropped along the way. Some practices have risen to the top and garnered uniform support. But it's not a perfect discipline. Like each case discussed in this book, the practice of social work needs to be reviewed from time to time. We need to question the practical application of certain principles in a changing world. If nothing else, the beauty of the social sciences is their fundamental concept that people are constantly changing. We need to remember this and embrace it.

LAST CLOSET DOOR

People with mental illnesses in our communities make up a huge part of our stigmatized populations. This is the last closet door that society has to open, accept, and embrace. There's a strong need to proactively find a way to provide meaningful services to this population.

After all, when we have a toothache, we go to the dentist. When it's an earache, we go to an ENT specialist. When we see someone who has a cut, we clean it and bandage it. When we see someone in a car accident, we call an ambulance. But when we feel depressed or stressed, what do we do? We ignore the symptoms and rely on hope to get better.

Every day, people we see around us are living with some form of mental illness, from anxiety disorder to depression to bipolar disorder or schizophrenia. It's estimated that one in five Americans has a form of mental illness. Yet, in most cases, we see nothing tangible so it's easy to forget about this population. But make no mistake, mental illness and its prevalence are real. Some call it the *next great epidemic* to face our nation and our world.

Stop and consider these numbers for the U.S., which is estimated to have a population of 325 million people in 2016: [1]

- *The health care costs in the U.S. are estimated at $3.55 trillion.* [2] *But money spent on mental illness represents just over one-hundredth of one percent (.014%) of that amount ($483 million).* [3]

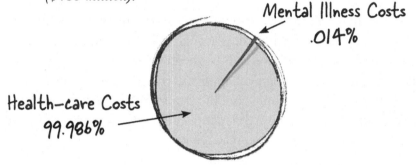

Mental Illness Costs
.014%

Health-care Costs
99.986%

THE PRISON POPULATION TODAY

A county in Florida wanting to alleviate overcrowding in its jails recognizes that the population of mentally ill people in jails and prisons is grossly overrepresented. Some estimate that, of the total population of prison inmates, fifteen to twenty percent are mentally ill or have a mental illness. The total population of American prisons is about two million, with approximately 340,000 people incarcerated who have a mental illness.[4] The cost of incarcerating a person with mental illness varies from $100,000 to $400,000 a year—a high price.

What if we could take half of that money and use it proactively to engage folks with mental illness in our communities?

What if we could stop cycling them through the criminal justice systems when their crimes are due more to illness than intentional criminal acts? Wouldn't implementing solutions to this dire situation be worth our efforts?

Consider this: One agency, Value Options Inc. in Connecticut, reports that in any six-month period, approximately 4,000 people will use psychiatric inpatient services in community-based hospitals, with the average length of stay being eight days. Most of these folks will be discharged to the same community setting that landed them in the hospital to begin with. They're put under the same faulty treatment plan with the same resources and overburdened public and private providers. The result? Nearly 160 will return in a week, and nearly 600 will return in a month!

What if this cycle were reduced by twenty-five percent? How much would this save?

LOOK AT THE COSTS

If private psychiatric units cost $1,000 a day (not to mention ambulance charges and other outside services), it could potentially cost $8,000 for one individual every two to three months! This means $32,000 a year for one person stuck in the revolving door of community-based living and involuntary commitment to a community hospital.

These numbers don't begin to consider the toll a mental illness takes on each individual. Likewise, they don't take into account the scars associated with each traumatic event that leads to hospitalization.

I've written this book to show how change can be accomplished. It's based on my experience in developing The Guardian Model as a powerful tool for community-based treatment across human services fields everywhere. This program is adaptable to children, people who are elderly, and developmentally disabled. It is simple, straightforward, and based on common sense. Its application is elementary, although I acknowledge that breaking habits and changing institutions is never easy. This is where out-of-the-box thinking comes in.

WHAT IS MELISSA'S PROJECT?

Since 2000, I have applied the principles of The Guardian Model in a program we call Melissa's Project. Its goal is to drastically reduce recidivism rates among individuals with mental illnesses. Specifically, it has recorded a twenty-five percent reduction in arrests among participants and an approximately seventy percent reduction in incarcerations. In communities using this model, overuse of private community hospitals has been reduced by nearly twenty-five percent and so has the number of patient admissions into hospital emergency departments.

On average, it costs about $6,000 a year for every participant in Melissa's Project. This is less than one eight-day stay at a private psychiatric hospital unit. The cost for 250 people to participate in this program is about $1.5 million.

The cost of incarcerating 250 individuals with mental illnesses is estimated, at best, at $25 million and, at worst, $100 million. The savings are estimated at $6 million based on the data collected that shows the reduction of arrests and incarcerations, ER usage, and stays in private and state psychiatric facilities. The numbers don't lie.

The value to people suffering with mental illnesses and struggling to break free of recidivism's revolving door should not be quantified. But in today's world, decisions made often come down to analyzing hard dollars. Who stops to consider how it will affect people tomorrow and well into the future?

It seems little thought is put into behavioral health issues which are treated like a side note to the broader discussions of popular health care. Yet if one in five people has a mental illness, for friends and families this issue can't be called a mere side note. It's an all-consuming reality of everyday life that won't go away with wishes.

Adopting The Guardian Model will help communities be

proactive and proficient in positively affecting lives in a large segment of our population.

I have filtered the successful traits of multiple systems providing care for individuals with mental illnesses and have discovered common characteristics that are demonstrated in the coming pages. I call these concepts 7 Cs, which make up the main ingredients for meaningfully delivering services to all populations in need.

The overarching principle in the book speaks to a concept of checks and balances known as Continuous Quality Improvement. Entire books and semesters at business schools are dedicated to understanding this concept. Here, I have broken it down to its core, showing how to conceptualize continuous quality improvement, simply and pragmatically.

Following that are examples of how to apply the 7 Cs to form the basis of good treatment. Consider it an introspective roadmap toward attaining Continuous Quality Improvement.

By using this book as your guide, you will learn to assist your clients in developing plans to improve their lives and your industry's ability to help them reach their goals. Let this book represent the starting line in the marathon to improved mental health systems or any Human Services in need of change.

CHAPTER 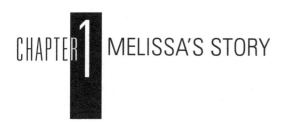1 MELISSA'S STORY

Melissa is confused. She is cold because she is miserably underdressed for the early winter weather. Where is her jacket? Where is her family? Are the men on the city green friends or threats?

Melissa is aware that, at some point, life changed. Her friends started to distance themselves from her. Even her best friend had had enough of Melissa's "attitude" and stopped returning her calls. Meanwhile, her mother became increasingly pushy and "all up in her business." Even her little sister seemed to be more and more intrusive or, alternatively, wanted nothing to do with her.

Then there were the doctors and the hospitals. Melissa can count six different hospitals in which she's been locked up. She's also vaguely aware of the fact that she's been in some hospitals more than once and that all of these stays took place over the last year or so. Why was everyone out to get her? Why would her mother place her in a hospital? Who the hell did that judge think he was anyhow? He doesn't know her!!

She approaches the men on the town common and sees that one of them is wearing her jacket. Why would that complete stranger have her jacket? Why are they smoking her cigarettes? Why are they laughing at her and talking about her? She can't control her anger and goes into a tirade demanding her jacket. Swearing, she aggressively confronts the group of men.

"Why are you laughing?" she screams, lunging for her jacket.

Melissa never sees the punch that leaves her unconscious, lying face down in the semi-frozen grass.

Melissa is a real person. Her life story symbolizes many others who suffer from mental illness, such as these individuals:

- *A twenty-four-year-old woman who has been involuntarily committed to at least nine different psychiatric facilities;*
- *A forty-five-year-old man who lives with schizophrenia, is addicted to crack cocaine and alcohol, and is repeatedly arrested for disorderly conduct;*
- *A thirty-three-year-old woman with bipolar disorder who is illiterate and prostitutes herself to support her drug habits;*
- *A thirty-seven-year-old man who, due to severe and persistent mental illness, believes he is a multimillionaire forced to live in poverty.*

Melissa also represents the following individuals:

- *A twenty-six-year-old woman with depression who wants to live independently, work, and attend college courses;*
- *A forty-year-old man who dreams of being an artist despite his severe mental illnesses;*
- *A twenty-seven-year-old man with schizophrenia who enjoys his job stocking shelves, listening to music, and socializing with his friends.*

Melissa has many faces but several characteristics in common with others. They include the following characteristics:

- *Severe and persistent mental illnesses;*
- *Involvement in the mental health system;*
- *Inability to make informed, rational decisions about activities of daily living;*
- *Mental health-care providers who have exhausted attempts to meet his/her needs;*
- *Involvement of several community-based treatment specialists;*
- *A desire to become involved with his/her own treatment;*

- *The will to live in the community;*
- *Personal goals, dreams, and desires.*

PEOPLE WITH MENTAL HEALTH ISSUES AND YOU

The lives of people with mental health issues are varied. Some are rich and fulfilled; others lack even the simplest of human needs. These individuals are as complex as all members of the general public. They rarely fit neatly within the client profile of any one state or local agency. Instead, most of them find themselves receiving services from many agencies, and quite often, the services or eligibility requirements of one may preclude services from another.

Now more than ever, the mental health system needs fresh approaches to effectively coordinate services among disparate providers and to deliver services to those with a mental illness who live in our communities.

Mental illness manifests itself in a number of ways. In some cases, illnesses are not obvious, and it's nearly impossible to tell that individuals have anything "wrong" with them. Others are so impaired that simple tasks such as showering, eating, and shopping present monumental obstacles every day.

Imagine your loved one is gravely ill. You have to take care of him or her, providing food, shelter, clothing. You would like this person to have a high quality of life with friends and social activities, work, and other means of fulfillment. Meanwhile, you need to work and care for the rest of your family. You want to ensure that this loved one—and you, too—have what's needed to make your lives meaningful and fulfilling.

Despite your best efforts to help your loved one, you are becoming increasingly frustrated because he or she simply doesn't get better. What's more, they act unpredictably and decompensate on a regular or increasing basis.

You realize you have to put your life on hold so you can continually respond to issues that face your loved one every day. Where would you begin? Do you know about state and local agencies that can help? Do you know about the courts specifically designed to address these types of needs?

THE LANGUAGE OF MENTAL ILLNESS

It's difficult to agree on appropriate terms to describe folks with mental illness. In fact, it's far easier to find consensus on what is *not* acceptable language.

After giving a presentation at a state psychiatric hospital, I received the following feedback: "You have a wonderful program, and as a speaker, you have much to offer people in need." It felt great to soak in that compliment. But then I heard this: "However, you need to learn to use more acceptable language that's not offensive to the population you are serving."

With that, I sought out my detractor and asked her to help me become more eloquent in language usage. I do not want to offend the people I seek to help! She graciously offered to send to my office a woman who would tell me about acceptable verbiage when discussing mental illness issues. Eager to hone my skills and my presentation, I graciously accepted.

I was surprised a few days later to meet a woman who was the most *un*-politically correct person I've ever met. She used words such as "crazy" and "nuts" and other phrases that would make anyone with sensibility uncomfortable. Then I learned this delightful pleasant woman herself has a mental illness. Perhaps she felt that gave her license to be un-PC.

Still, from her, I learned one phrase that I've used ever since: "Persons with mental illnesses." I can't begin to say how many times I was told this sounds ridiculous and grammatically incorrect. But out of deference and loyalty to my new ally, I stuck with it for fifteen years until another mental health advocacy group admonished me. People in this group contended that the phrase "mental illnesses" suggests all folks have more than one illness.

In addition, I was told not to use the word "consumer" because it implies people have choice when it comes to mental illnesses. On top of that, a well-known psychiatrist and mental health activist told me he prefers to be called a "schizophrenic" rather than "a person living with schizophrenia"!

It's hard to be PC. I do my best.

Throughout these pages, you'll see various terms used interchangeably without any intent to offend. At times, I call people "clients" and "participants" when referring to their role within a system of care. Those who come to my practice are not my "patients," as I'm not a doctor; I'm an attorney.

As an attorney, my mandate is to follow my clients' directions. I am ethically bound to serve their interests in terms of what they want. This is often in juxtaposition to what they may need or find in their best interest.

This is the beauty of the Human Services fields; practitioners are bound to act in a clients' best interest. Perhaps it's this "best interest standard" that passionately brings me to this field as I focus on fixing issues that prevent service delivery efficiently and effectively.

About the language to use, I prefer to call people with mental illnesses "individuals." This blanket term reminds us that all people are unique and that their care should be as well. That said, when individuals are in a program, I refer to them as "participants." It indicates they have the free will to partake in planning and be an integral part of the team process. Similarly, they have the free will to exclude themselves.

No matter what we call people with mental illnesses, they are, in fact, people who have dreams and hopes and desires like every one of us.

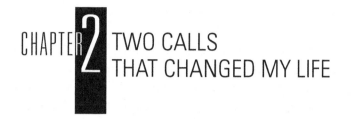

CHAPTER 2 TWO CALLS THAT CHANGED MY LIFE

The practice of law is not the stuff of TV or film. Although it's often called "a profession," it isn't glamorous. In fact, it's become little more than a tough business. Practitioners are typically not paid the salaries made famous in fairy tales. They have tremendously high student loans and are beholden to the calendars of others, making life stressful, frantic, and unhealthy. A solo practitioner is lowest on the totem pole. The guy or gal who is working in the probate field focused on mental incapacity, conservatorships, and guardianships is the lowliest of the low.

That's me.

Somehow, I decided it would be great to walk out of law school, hang a shingle, and peddle my wares to every probate court within a thirty-minute drive of my office/house. Probate courts are always looking for attorneys to represent indigent folks in matters pertaining to child custody and mental health, or anyone who hasn't the means to obtain counsel on their own. Naturally, the rate of pay for this service is drastically reduced so a lawyer in this situation has to take on a great deal of work to keep the lights on.

My interests pulled me to represent people under conservatorship (called guardianship in some states). These are adults who are in need of third-party representation to make informed decisions about their day-to-day care and finances. The reason for the appointment can be anything from dementia to severe mental illness, victimization to reckless expenditures.

As I said, it's not glamorous. At the time I started doing this work, the rate of pay was set at a maximum of $250 a year for individuals residing in a facility and $500 for those living in the community. I hoped that for every five of these cases, I'd land on one that could be parlayed into something substantial.

Within a few short years, I had accumulated more than a hundred files of this sort, and my life was complete chaos. While I struggled to keep up with the demands of other business—real estate closings, evictions, personal injury files—the fiduciary files fell to the bottom of the pile. They're simply low on the list of priorities because, after all, one needs to eat.

This state of affairs was unsettling to me, someone who lies awake at night brooding about things. My conservator files ate at me. Where was Joe? Did Emily get discharged from the hospital? Did Billy get his medications delivered?

Add to that the fact that a phone call to a lawyer's office is never good. I can count on one hand the numbers of times I've received a call that didn't present a problem. Likewise, the mail rarely contains a check. My practice, like that of many of my colleagues, became the perfect example of "no news is good news." So I became reactive, jumping from fire to fire, never realizing I was the "arsonist" who set the blaze.

That was true until I was lucky enough to find a niche—or the niche found me.

I have received two phone calls that changed my life. One was from Melissa's mom and the other from the local probate court.

MY PARADIGM SHIFT

Let me start with an important premise, a monumental paradigm shift. It's this: *Under an effective system of care, we should not begin by considering what a person is incapable of doing. Rather, we should start our inquiry with the person's capabilities and use compassionate decision making to fill in the gaps.*

That means instead of looking at problems, an effective system of care should look at what the person *can* do and build from that. This paradigm is based on a "person-centered" approach, and everything grows from there.

But first, let me describe the two calls I received.

THE FIRST CALL

The call was fairly straightforward. A friend was on the line telling me to get to the hospital because a family desperately needed my help.

At the time, I had been practicing law for ten years. I had a reputation as a no-nonsense lawyer who wasn't afraid to identify and talk frankly about the issues facing his clients. So, without trepidation, I made my way to the hospital to meet with a woman who would change my life—and the lives of thousands of others.

As I walked down the main hall of the hospital's psychiatric unit, I heard a heated conversation coming from a conference room. The friend who had phoned me earlier was on the receiving end of a tirade from another woman. This second woman was not so subtly dancing around the belief that my friend, the hospital, and the entire city were inept beyond compare. Her daughter's issues, she declared, were a direct result of their shortcomings.

After my friend de-escalated this emotional situation, I learned this other woman was named Robin. Her ire was based on the hospital's inability to determine what was wrong with her daughter Melissa. It seemed there was no plan to address the issues facing Melissa and her family.

Because of privacy issues and Melissa being over the age of eighteen, necessarily and legally Robin was told very little about her daughter's care.

I tried my best to get a story from Robin that made sense. Angry and in a great deal of emotional pain, she sensed she was losing her loved one, her baby. The girl she knew was becoming a stranger to her and her family.

Sadly, the story she told me next is one I've heard many times over the years.

A FAMILY'S STRUGGLE

Melissa was Robin's golden child, outgoing, kind, ambitious, and wise beyond her years. She was popular in school and had good grades. She had a strong work ethic and a tight group of friends. Even her younger sister would admit Melissa was the one most likely to go places in life. She had worked at a local pharmacy since she was fifteen years old and was the darling of the town where they lived.

Things began to change for Melissa as she grew apart from her mother and sister and fell in with "the wrong crowd." Her grades slipped and her childhood friends fell by the wayside. She dabbled a bit in drugs and alcohol and began missing work often.

After graduating from high school, she distanced herself further from her loved ones. She disappeared for long periods in an irresponsible fashion, not allowing friends or family to know her whereabouts. She returned home only when she needed money or a bath or both.

Robin became angry and Melissa's sister became worried, scared, and sad. This was not the girl they had known for nineteen years.

Melissa continued to slide and couldn't hold down a job. She lost all her friends. In the rare moments she did speak to her mother and sister, her tone was irate, short, and distant. She pushed them further and further away. Her absences from home increased in duration as well as frequency.

Reaching out to local mental health providers offered little relief for this family. For those of means, services are readily accessible in the community. However, these resources are typically not comprehensive and have little structure or continuity of care.

Conversely, public mental health systems are designed to be comprehensive in the services they offer. Unfortunately, enrolling in these systems is cumbersome.

No matter where one finds oneself on the economic spectrum, knowledge of which mental health services are available is extremely limited. Further, little guidance exists concerning what best fits the needs of a particular individual. This is due to dozens of factors, from cognitive functioning to geographic locale.

Lying awake every night, Robin would hope for a phone call from a distant hospital or emergency room saying Melissa was there safe in the confines of their walls. And in a six-month period, these calls came nine times—from Hartford, Connecticut, to Harrisburg, Pennsylvania.

Frustrations mounted as, time after time, Melissa was discharged after a brief hospitalization. She would return to the community and her patterns of behavior. These same patterns resulted in further trauma for Melissa as well as desperate worry for her mother.

Premature discharge from a hospital is a direct cause of, and potentially less productive than, repeated hospitalizations. When Melissa is discharged without thoughtful planning, she's being set up for failure. What follows is the inevitable trauma of decompensations and its potentially dangerous consequences to her and the community.

Prior to our conversation in the hospital, Robin hadn't seen Melissa for ten days. The police had found her unconscious behind the city library on a cold November day. They described her as unresponsive and near death, severely beaten and left without a coat to shield her against the cold winter night.

WHAT MELISSA'S STORY
MEANS TO HUMAN SERVICES PROFESSIONALS

As a professional in Human Services, how many "Melissas" do you know? How many "Melissas" have you watched spiral around your system of care while their families agonized over them? How many times have you wanted to do more but felt hamstrung by the limitations of your role? Have you ever watched as others neglected to perform duties integral to the success of your "Melissas"?

This story illustrates the frustrations facing caregivers who struggle to make their way through human service systems. Like Melissa, they themselves

- *are struggling for independence,*
- *are coping with a disease that's crippling the essence of that independence,*
- *have visited multiple hospitals across geographic regions that don't communicate with each other,*
- *are involved in a system of care that remains a mystery, available but somehow out of reach to those who need it most,*
- *have angry families who can't understand the illness or its manifestations, nor why they can't find the help they so desperately need, and*
- *are part of a family that's grieving their "loss."*

In retelling this story, Robin reaffirmed what I'd already seen in practice: Human Services Systems are often dysfunctional, fragmented, inefficient, and above all dismissive.

STATE OF THE INDUSTRY

The Human Services industry is limping along, trying to keep up with budget cuts, ever-changing social issues, and negative perceptions. Yet this industry affects needy and vulnerable citizens every second of every day.

The challenges facing individuals in need aren't limited to mental illness; they span the spectrum of developmental disabilities, children's issues, and eldercare.

Like many of my colleagues, I stayed awake that night pondering how to help Melissa and Robin, Billy and Emily, and the dozens of others I'm obligated to assist under the weight of every fiduciary code ever written. If only I'd known then what I know now!

THE SECOND CALL

I mentioned my late night broodings to a prominent probate judge. He was quite concerned with the plight of folks with mental illnesses residing in his jurisdiction. He supported me wholeheartedly and introduced me to a nurse to "flesh out" my ideas for change. This first meeting didn't amount to much, but the seed had been cast and, several months later, I received another momentous phone call.

As usual, I dreaded picking up the phone. I was even more alarmed when I was summoned to the judge's chambers for a "talk." (Lawyers don't get called to judge's chambers just to talk.) So, after taking an extra dose of my anxiety medication, I set out to see what I'd gotten myself into.

As it turned out, Judge Lawlor had been in serious discussion with the medical director of the Connecticut Department of Mental Health, Dr. Ken Marcus. The two were likeminded in their concern over the extraordinary rates of recidivism at local and state emergency rooms and hospitals.

Judge Lawlor asked if I was still operating my "project" and what I needed to make it work. The short answer, of course, was "I need money." The long answer, which I gave then and continue to give, is that I simply needed an audience.

First, people must be made aware of the issues people in the conservator/guardianship field face daily. Then we can come together with realistic resolutions for a better system of care. In turn, this will result in the reduction of recidivism, better informed systems, proactive approaches, and greater efficiency. Most important, it will bring overall increases in empowerment and life satisfaction to those we represent.

Judge Lawlor and Dr. Marcus lent me their credibility and secured me an audience—several audiences, in fact. They also committed themselves, trusting that their respective systems, Probate Courts and Mental Health Services, should and could do a better job for the at-need populations they serve. Fortuitously, Judge Lawlor was soon named the probate court administrator for the state of Connecticut.

In 2001, a steering committee was formed consisting of representatives from Connecticut's Probate Court Administration, the Department of Mental Health, the Chief Forensic Psychiatrist's Office, and Yale University, plus my partner/clinical director, Sara Valentino, and me. Our mission was to develop a plan for the efficient delivery of services to individuals with severe, persistent mental illnesses in the community. This was truly a collaborative dialogue to stop the "revolving door" experienced by this population.

The 2001 steering committee discussed the "real" issues facing practitioners in the Human Services field every day. For one, courts don't understand the needs of community-based providers, while those providers don't understand the needs of inpatient settings and so on. Public providers are altogether unique and have an entirely different set of needs than their private counterparts. Systems of care are horribly fragmented, which causes those most in need to fall through the cracks. This results in repeated visits to emergency rooms and jails. What is that costing in money and human suffering?

These meetings gave birth to concepts that have been developed into The Guardian Model. This book introduces you to those innovative concepts. More than that, it shows how you can use them daily as you make profound changes to your agency and the field of Human Services itself.

Under The Model, the goal is the creation of an Interrelated

System of Care. As mentioned earlier, there are common characteristics or "personality traits" of an Interrelated System of Care that I call the 7 Cs.

The Guardian Model compels practitioners to develop plans that consider 7 Cs in all facets. Thereafter, The Model asks them to continually and proactively review the plan created, preferably applying the seven essential elements—7 Cs.

The next chapter takes a deeper look at the value of developing an interrelated service system of care.

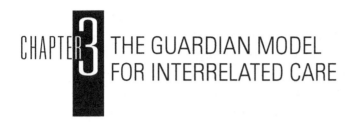

CHAPTER 3 THE GUARDIAN MODEL
FOR INTERRELATED CARE

The elements of a good service system are quite basic. However, changing systems that have been in place for decades is like pushing a glacier uphill. Technically speaking, the concepts are simple, but the practical application across disparate providers and institutions is extremely difficult. The first move is to create what I call a system of care that's interrelated, as defined here.

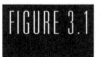

Interrelated: having an interdependent or intergrated connection between two or more entities that maximizes potential for all

Certain ingredients are critical to every interrelated system, which I refer to as 7 Cs. They operate most effectively when they're interdependent and mixed with the proper dash of ambition, introspection, and daring.

The 7 Cs, described in Chapter Four, combine to create a massive eighth C known as Continuous Quality Improvement (CQI). This is a fancy way of saying *a system will implement its own process of checks and balances to protect against complacency and apathy while ensuring it's proactive in providing treatment.* These frequent checks make sure clients don't fall through the cracks of the system, and they continue to have their needs met.

Think of this eighth C—CQI—as the destination where we want to be under all Interrelated Service Systems. In action, CQI becomes a living entity. It changes, morphing where it needs to, growing and contracting and healing itself by its very nature. A wise person once said, "When we continuously improve, the next thing we do will be the greatest thing we've ever done."

I don't believe in change for the sake of change. Change is never easy, and it would not be here. But the tools for change are readily available to each of us.

I will be the first to acknowledge that, if systems worked the way they're supposed to, I wouldn't have a job and you wouldn't be reading this book. But I know that we walk on common ground in our acceptance that systems today do *not* function effectively. They can always be more efficient, which is why the concepts for change are within your reach. It's a disservice to those most at need to continue the dysfunction we have collectively allowed to develop.

That said, implementing a better system of care isn't as difficult as it sounds. It can be accomplished by sheer force of will and commitment on the part of a relatively small number of folks ready to make changes on a massive scale. Many of us in the field are motivated because we're angry at what's around us. This system provides a model for ways to ensure quality services to the populations we care about the most.

BENEFITS OF
AN INTERRELATED SYSTEM OF CARE

Think of it this way. If I do my job well and you do yours well and everyone else at the table does the same, at least three benefits will emerge:

- *Everyone's job will feel easier.*
- *We will work collaboratively in a more efficient manner.*
- *Our mutual clients will benefit from our efficiency and the resulting attention we can give to their needs.*

The ideal characteristics of an Interrelated Service System are threefold:

1. *Realistic and attainable treatment plans.*

2. *Positive relationships.*

3. *Empowerment.*

Let's examine each of these.

1. Realistic and attainable treatment plans.

A plan for the sake of having a plan is a waste of time and an insult to the very people we are planning for. There's no sense in dusting off a plan that was shown to be shortsighted and unsuccessful in the hopes of skipping difficult work and cutting corners. It's a travesty to send people into the community with a treatment plan that has proven its ineffectiveness and landed individuals in the hospital due to one or more key failures. Considering the trauma associated with repeated decompensation and hospitalization, it borders on unethical. It's frustrating, duplicative, duplicitous, and inefficient, not to mention traumatic for the individual involved. We need to do the things we say we will and try new things that may not have been tried before.

2. Positive relationships.

This system promotes collaborative measures with service providers in the community and disseminates important information to appropriate authorized individuals while utilizing a strengths-based ecological approach.

We all work *for* our mutual client, *not* the other way around. We have to "play nice in the sandbox," talk to each other, and share what's available to us.

Unfortunately, there's a tendency to be possessive of information and resources in bureaucracies. People climb all over each other to gain credit or escape blame for the circumstances of those served. This is maddening because the resources I refer to are generally provided by taxpayer dollars. Therefore, they belong to all of us and we, as a society, have directed providers to use them for the benefit of the public in need.

Naturally, we can't go around sharing everyone's business with whomever we want due to issues of privacy. However, I don't encourage anyone to hide behind the Health Insurance Portability and Accountability Act of 1996 (HIPAA) as a reason for a breakdown in communication or collaboration.

3. Empowerment.

When individuals are better informed about treatment, medications, and options available to them, they feel more capable of controlling aspects of daily life. They report more involvement in community, social, and family settings. They feel empowered to determine the course of treatment and their participation therein.

Empowerment is everything. We can't expect a treatment plan or a discharge plan to work when we don't include the subject of that plan in its making. I can't even count the number of times I've been at the table with a huge team of players representing various components of a treatment plan. We're supposed to gather regularly to discuss a plan we created as a team in the past and tweak it where appropriate. We also need to set goals for our mutual client. However, the client is the one person not in attendance.

I can sit here all day making plans and setting goals for Melissa. But if she isn't a part of these grand schemes, they *will* fail. She must be invested in them. She has to direct me and the entire team about where she wants to go. We are the crew; she is the captain. So she has to set the course and destination, and it's our job to take her there. This is why The Guardian Model is so successful.

OUTCOMES OF AN INTERRELATED SERVICE SYSTEM

Under an Interrelated Service System, we can expect the following measurable outcomes:

- *Fiscal responsibility and efficiency*
- *Resource sharing among disparate agencies and providers*
- *Reduction in recidivism in the medical, legal, and civil processes*
- *Increased client participation, empowerment, and trust*
- *Appropriate allocation of responsive interventions among disparate agencies and providers*
- *Proactive approaches to treatment and discharge planning*

In addition, the following qualitative outcomes are possible:

- *Clients agree they are better informed about their illness, treatment, medications, and options available to them.*
- *Clients feel they've been empowered to determine the course of treatment and participants.*
- *Clients feel more capable of controlling aspects of their daily living.*
- *Clients show more participation in community, social, and family settings.*

Just saying we want all these great things won't make it so. The 7 Cs, described in the next chapter, give us the roadmap to nurture this interrelatedness. Once we've arrived there, the efficiency of our work will be astounding.

EXPLAINING HIPAA

The Health Insurance Portability and Accountability Act of 1996 was enacted primarily to help folks keep health insurance by ensuring that certain entities are not allowed to share potentially damaging information about an individual. It's in place to protect the individual, not the agency or insurance company that provides services.

The part of the law we tend to forget about is that *it permits the disclosure of health information needed for patient care and other important purposes.*

In addition to service providers hiding behind client choice, free will, and the right to make bad decisions, many institutions and agencies take a rigid stance on information sharing. These entities claim that patient confidentiality is protected by HIPAA. However, there's a big difference between standard privacy rights and the scope of HIPAA.

Wearing my lawyer hat, let me state that HIPAA does not apply when team members are working under an identified treatment plan for the best interest of a mutual client, particularly in emergency situations.

HIPAA has rarely been actionable in courts of law, and awards for violations of HIPAA involving health-care professionals have rarely been given, if ever. Almost invariably, if the question arises, "Does HIPAA apply here?" the answer is "no."

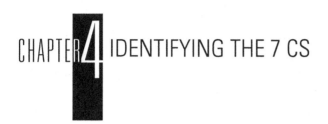

CHAPTER 4 IDENTIFYING THE 7 CS

The 7 Cs make up a large part of your Human Services toolbox. Let's look at what they are and why they're important.

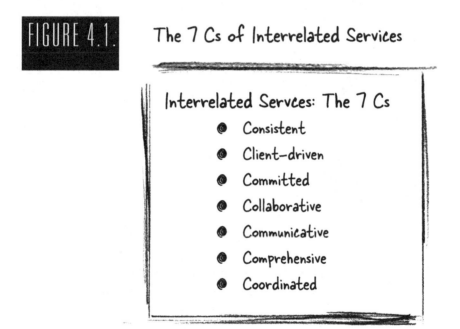

FIGURE 4.1. The 7 Cs of Interrelated Services

Interrelated Servces: The 7 Cs
- Consistent
- Client-driven
- Committed
- Collaborative
- Communicative
- Comprehensive
- Coordinated

For a system of care to become interrelated, those involved must be willing to evolve and to adopt the characteristics of the 7 Cs listed in Figure 4.1. In doing so, providers necessarily impact change on a broad spectrum internally, which perpetuates change across service systems as a whole.

As you look at this list of 7 Cs, consider each of them as more than words. They're not policies or procedures, nor are they boilerplate concepts. They are seven *calls to action*. Although they're adjectives, treat them as if they were action verbs to inspire and guide you on what to do to serve your clients successfully. These 7 Cs will form the foundation for your thought process as you use these "actions" to assess needs and resources on a case-by-case basis.

~

To illustrate each of the 7 Cs, let's follow the story of Jeffrey. It explains how each of the 7 Cs plays a vital role in the delivery of services to him and other people in need.

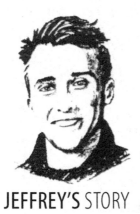

JEFFREY'S STORY

By the time he was seventeen, Jeffrey had a psychiatric diagnosis of schizoaffective disorder and a history of huffing (sniffing glue) from a young age. He had burned every bridge he'd crossed.

I met Jeffrey after being appointed as his conservator of person. When he was added to my caseload, Jeffrey had been treated psychiatrically in several different areas of the state and was struggling mightily to maintain life in the community. He was young and wanted to be "normal." He wanted a girlfriend and buddies.

He wanted to party like a twenty-something and live a life similar to those around him. But Jeffrey's persistent mental illness was a problem. Plus, he'd seriously damaged his brain cells and was cognitively compromised. Operating with insufficient insight, he wanted nothing to do with services being offered by various mental health providers.

I admit I was in a "no news is good news mode" at the time, so Jeffrey's neediness was overwhelming to me as well as to his providers. We all breathed a sigh of relief when he was moved to a catchment area on the far side of the state. There he would be given a new team.

As luck (or fate) would have it, he turned out to be one of the first clients assigned to my new program, Melissa's Project, because his failure to use the services offered continued to be a source of frustration and even irritation.

When we "picked him up," Jeffrey had been involuntarily committed to a psychiatric hospital. Because he desperately wanted to return to his hometown thirty miles to the north, one day while on a cigarette break, he simply walked away. No news was no longer good news.

A day or so after walking away, Jeffrey was arrested for creating a public disturbance. The police found him on the town green screaming at a light pole. When he was processed at the police station, it turned out he had a few outstanding warrants, which meant he'd be staying with the local authorities for a while. Or so I thought.

My memory is a bit foggy, but one thing is clear to me: I've never seen the criminal justice system move with such speed or efficiency. Before long, Jeffrey was placed in a high security prison, which allegedly had a strong mental health component. To be arrested and summarily incarcerated is bad enough. But imagine being arrested after escaping from a psychiatric institution for exhibiting symptoms of the mental illness that placed you there to begin with. Simply absurd.

It became my number one priority to get this poor kid back to the hospital where he had a chance of receiving targeted mental health treatment.

GATHERING A TEAM

To that end, we made several phone calls attempting to get Jeffrey out of jail. We scheduled a meeting and somehow managed to get chief players to the table. The social worker from the Public Defender's office was there to relay our plans to the criminal courts. A representative from Court Support Services (CSS) attended because that group had ultimate control of probation and assigning jurisdiction to the courts. A representative from Jail Diversion was present to discuss options regarding Jeffrey's pending charges. Representatives of the Department of Mental Health brought to the table available resources that could be committed to Jeffrey's care if he were returned to the psychiatric hospital. Of course, I was present as his fiduciary, and I brought my partner and cofounder, Sara, whom I introduced to the team as my Care Coordinator, a term that was not being used in 2001. By her presence, I wanted her to be accepted as a valuable team member who would relay important information back to me and ensure that Jeffrey would feel comfortable with her.

Having these people in the room from so many vital disciplines caused me to realize for the first time the pure power in what we had set out to do. This type of gathering was a game changer that would benefit Jeffrey and countless others.

CSS started to talk to the public defender's office about realistic placement options. The prosecutor wasn't represented so they had to speculate about what would be palatable not only to the judge but also to the "state." Mental Health representatives chimed in with their own promises and commitment to ensure, above all else, Jeffrey's safety. Sara and I offered our commitment to follow up and keep all the parties informed of progress in the case. After an hour of candid discussions about resources, limitations, and an overabundance of acronyms and legal jargon, we had a plan to get Jeffrey out of jail and back to the hospital.

PLANNING TO PLAN

Did you notice an interesting issue with this story? We had to "plan to plan" here. Before we could even get down to the work of looking at Jeffrey's case, we had to first remove all kinds of barriers to his treatment, such as imprisonment, transportation, and securing an appropriate bed.

This illustrates that while I can break down the review of a service system the players may change, but the underlying problems facing the system remain. As with an onion, you can peel away layers that are rotting, but when you get to the core, it's still an onion, and it still smells.

For instance, the police had no way of knowing that Jeffrey had been involuntarily committed to a hospital by a court of proper jurisdiction. They didn't know (although it should have been obvious) that Jeffrey suffered from a mental illness and his actions were the manifestation of that illness. The result, his yelling at a light pole, was not of willful criminality.

In addition, no one had called to inform the police Jeffrey had eloped from the psychiatric unit and would likely show up in town. The conservator received no information about Jeffrey's whereabouts until he was locked up.

HAPPY RESULTS

Jeffrey did get back to the hospital. The judge was advised by the public defender's office that we had coordinated a meeting and put a comprehensive plan in place to ensure Jeffrey's safety and the safety of the community. The judge was satisfied. Eventually, the prosecutor, seeing that much was being done for Jeffrey's benefit, agreed to hold Jeffrey's other charges in abeyance.

What would have happened had I not been involved? Would Jeffrey have stayed in prison? Would he have received adequate mental health treatment? Would he have decompensated while incarcerated and acted out, earning him a longer stay?

COMPONENTS OF THE 7 CS

Since I met Jeffrey, I've consulted on hundreds of cases with variations of the same themes. In these cases, certain patterns continued to develop and I noticed that plans worked best when they shared common characteristics. I call these beneficial traits the 7Cs. Any case and any system that truly wants to be efficient and effective should demonstrate consideration of these seven elements.

An explanation of each component of the 7 Cs follows.

1. CONSISTENT

Systems of care need to demonstrate *consistency* on both a macro and a micro level. People working in the system must be consistent. This constitutes the micro level. The same workers should be working with the same people and families for a prolonged period.

However, Human Services fields suffer from a high turnover, and frequent personnel change is never good for seamless application of care. Clients need to gain a comfort level with providers, which is appropriate and necessary to a successful clinical relationship. Participants also have the right to hold certain expectations that those they've built relationships and trust with will consistently work for their benefit.

On a macro level, consistency is critical in ensuring that once a program has demonstrated willingness to move toward interrelatedness, it will not veer from this path. Service providers make this promise to each other in the spirit of collaboration, with the understanding that we are interrelated. Therefore, we all depend on each other to influence the change we want to see. The message is made clear to staff and other providers: *The most critical members of the treatment team accept the challenges of interrelatedness.* They foresee the value to all and to their mutual clients, and they're willing to ride out the difficulties inherent in its application.

In Jeffrey's case, I provided consistency by following up with all the representatives to ensure their piece of the plan was put into action. I also openly discussed the efficacy of their efforts and their limitations.

2. COMMITTED

Interrelatedness doesn't come easy to long-established systems of care. It's vital to the success of these systems to be consistent in approach (the first C) and committed to stay the course despite many bumps in the road. The most functional systems are committed to this change and understand that the results of interrelatedness far outweigh the discomfort of getting there.

The change starts from the top with this insight: "We can, and should, be doing a better job for our clients." Administrators need to be willing to say they aren't happy with the work product they've designed. Then the staff members in the system need to feel they're supported in a quest to constantly do more and do it better.

However, in practice, it's quite often a "trickle up" phenomenon, in which the impetus for real change is the frustration and anger felt by direct-care staff on a day-to-day basis. The discontent of the line staff is quite often the first indication to management that change is not only warranted but also vital.

The people who showed up at the table that day were committed to Jeffrey's case. This was particularly true because we were all familiar with him and knew jail wasn't where he should be. Each person offered his or her time and expertise to find a resolution, recognizing the alternative would be seriously detrimental to Jeffrey's progress and eventual release to the community.

3. COLLABORATIVE

CSS was willing to work with the public defender to do what was in Jeffrey's best interest. All others were willing to work with me as the fiduciary representative to ensure Jeffrey's safety and appropriate care. Although representatives of the prosecutor's office and court weren't in the room, the group also acknowledged the importance of representing their interest in the spirit of this collaboration to ensure a positive outcome.

Interrelated systems of care collaborate. People share ideas and successes and failures. They're willing to open themselves up to criticism and grow with the support of disparate providers who may have a different, if not better, means of attaining similar goals.

Collaboration is difficult, although it receives lip service when agency heads and politicos compete for publicity around a vow to work together. What matters are the true nuts and bolts of the collaboration that go on behind closed doors. Collaboration doesn't happen in a vacuum. It's often the byproduct of difficult and often embarrassing admissions of shortcomings as well as frank requests for the assistance of others.

Such introspection and transparency can be scary and often painful. We can feel embarrassed by our own and our agency's "failures." And the not-for-profit sector is constantly looking over its collective shoulder, worrying about funding and competition for scarce dollars.

That said, the result is well worth the turmoil of the process, and the positive change far outweighs the individual fears people feel when participating in the journey. We're all in it together.

An important insight: *I may fail today and you may fail tomorrow, but the important thing is we pick each other up and carry on.*

4. COMMUNICATIVE

It was fun to watch the energy in the room as the agency representatives bandied about different programs and acronyms for resources at their disposal that might work in Jeffrey's case. Although the conversation was hard to follow at times, it was open and candid. The participants discussed system shortcomings and offered suggestions. We saw how positive energy can be born out of common purpose and a feeling of community and like-mindedness.

There are many different ways to think about communication. On the one hand, we can look at the manner in which we communicate with clients, such as an impersonal telephone call, e-mail, and texts or a person-to-person meeting in which engagement and relationship building are part of the focus of treatment.

Beyond this, institutionalized descriptors for communication can hamstring providers and their ability to engage in meaningful conversation outside of their particular agency. Indeed, some institutional cultures prescribe minimal communication *inside* the walls of their own offices.

Of course, it's vital we gather information, but perhaps the key to an efficient system is sharing or disseminating the information that we gather. Information must flow seamlessly and must be reliable.

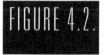 Information Flow from Provider to Provider

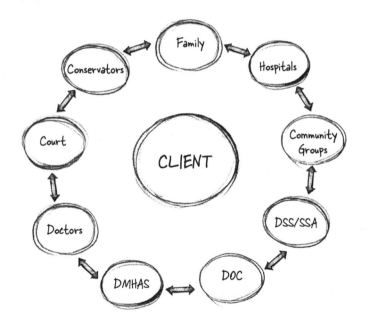

How many times has a representative from a nursing agency arrived to administer medication only to learn that the patient was hospitalized overnight? How often do delivery services fail to show up to transport a client to a doctor's appointment? How often are doctors' appointments miscommunicated between offices to clients or other providers? And how many times have we endured the death of a client due to contraindicated medications to treat different maladies? It has happened in my practice, and one time is too many.

5. COMPREHENSIVE

The team didn't hold back in its commitment to bring together resources and make Jeffrey's transition back to the hospital as seamless as possible. CSS pulled the strings necessary to get him released from jail. The public defender spoke to the prosecutor and the court about the need for this to happen. The Department of Mental Health made sure Jeffrey's bed would be available for him upon release from jail. Sara and I coordinated transportation and facilitated the conversation to transfer medications and records between facilities before and after his discharge.

Do you see how interrelatedness depends on the system of providers being "all in"? It relies on the assumption that the treatment team is a group of providers seeking the same goal: *the best interest of our mutual client.* Therefore, we must be certain that our commitment extends to a belief in the value of creating an interrelated system. We also need to trust participants to bring to bear, in every case, all they have in their arsenal of goods and services.

This isn't about holding back or wanting to horde what is "mine." It's a concept that all of your resources and all of my resources are "ours," and we can avail ourselves of them freely, openly, and honestly.

Indeed, resources at our disposal as care providers aren't truly "ours." We hold them in trust until such time as they're used to benefit our clients. It's not unlike a fiduciary responsibility we have and, as such, we are mandated to employ our resources responsibly whenever appropriate and necessary.

6. CLIENT-DRIVEN

In our society, we've wandered far from the basic concept that systems exist only because our mutual clients allow us to exist and not the other way around. Once we establish this as a basic tenet, it's easier to allow—even encourage—clients to be empowered to take a real stake in their own treatment. In a client-driven system of care, the wishes, hopes, and desires of the client should draw the chart that assists the team in navigating the ship through potentially rough seas.

Note I said the "the team." The client is an essential *participant* of the team. The health services team is *not* in charge of the patient—quite the opposite. Our clients inform us of their goals, as noted by the arrows in Figure 4.3 coming outwardly from the middle.

The arrows going back to the middle represent what each member of the treatment team can give to assist the person in achieving the goals she or he has set. It's no small coincidence that this model is set up like a diagram of a solar system. In it, all of the moving parts are inextricably pulled in and around the center focal point of the system.

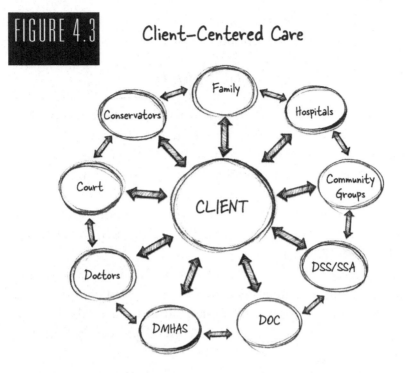

FIGURE 4.3   Client-Centered Care

7. COORDINATED

This meeting about Jeffrey and thousands more have taken place because we, an independent third party, took time to alert the appropriate parties of major issues. We balanced the busy schedules of the major players and facilitated a meeting, drafted an agenda, and identified the core issues for the team. To the extent necessary, we served as a proctor for the meeting and kept its focus so we could come up with a realistic and attainable plan within a limited time frame.

This final C is perhaps the most instrumental because it sets an interrelated service system apart from all others. An interrelated service system uses an independent third party as a monitoring, reporting, and coordinating entity. In turn, this Care Coordinator ensures ongoing good-faith participation of all team members. Often, this person is the unwelcome guest at the dinner table (at least until the other parties see what that guest brought for dessert). It's human nature to question the credibility and relevance of a newcomer. When that newcomer asks questions of a team or gathers detailed information to shed light on issues affecting treatment, he or she may be seen as an outlier quite quickly.

Under The Guardian Model, Sara became the first Care Coordinator. Her role was to be both a cheerleader and a coxswain in the back of the boat, redirecting the team on its straight and even path.

Again, it's vital for management to understand that we strive for a uniform level of performance across the team. Each piston must fire to make the engine run. The Care Coordinator assures all of the other moving parts that they can rely upon this basic fact of operation. And make no mistake; it can be as hot and uncomfortable as a combustion engine when the coordinator of care, observing from the outside, points out flaws in the plan or identifies where one component is not fulfilling its obligations to the rest.

In addition to the seven most important ingredients of interrelated services, let's not forget Compassion. Compassion brought people into the industry to begin with, and I'm hoping to reconnect you to that compassion.

Cash is often something providers have no control over, and I choose to deal with elements we can individually and collectively change. I can't change the fiscal morass of the world economy. But my systems were just as strapped for cash when we began this process as are all of yours.

There's no need for limitless resources when we implement the model I'm describing here. Resources are and will always be limited. But, using this simple structure, starting with an understanding of the 7 Cs, will allow any system to implement positive growth.

These seven ingredients combined in seven to the seventh power give us more than 820,000 possible combinations to tackle any problem that may come up.

These 820,000 possible combinations create a wonderfully flexible pool from which to draw. I think of all 7 Cs each time

I'm consulting on a difficult case. In some instances, I use a table-spoon of Comprehensive and a dash of Collaboration with a cup of Consistent. Other times, I need a pound of Collaboration and a pinch of Communication to direct the team. This is the power of the program, and using the combination of principles in the model I'm offering gives you a universe of tools at your disposal. The biggest and most important tool of all is coming next. Trust me, you'll need a bigger toolbox.

Look back on this and understand the magnitude of this example for your agency and the folks you represent. The most difficult aspect is Coordination; it deals with scheduling busy people across disparate services in different parts of the state. But once the meeting is coordinated, you'll have set in motion the mecha-nism that allows providers to bring their expertise to the table. It truly takes on a life of its own in most circumstances.

When the right questions are asked in the spirit of collabora-tion, when the right challenges are posed and exposed in the spirit of communication, when the right promises are made in the spirit of consistency and commitment, plans create themselves. Hope-fully, they do so in a client-driven manner. After that, it's up to you to constantly foster the plan's application, which is what Chapter Five tackles.

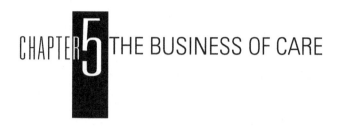

CHAPTER 5 THE BUSINESS OF CARE

The idea of Continuous Quality Improvement (CQI) is age-old in the business sector. It's a simple principle that more or less means we need to double-check our work. Scholars have gone out of their way for years, however, to make it more complicated than this. Some CQI models are extremely complicated and can be even more cumbersome than the job they purport to review. Naturally, I prefer to take an easier approach as I explain my own version of CQI in this chapter.

By definition, CQI requires that a designated party (Care Coordinator) monitor and report on the process developed. This component keeps everyone else "honest" and dedicated to the process. Of course, *influencing* the participation of providers proves more effective than coercion in order to achieve cooperation.

CQI is an initiative implemented by staff, encouraged by management, and welcomed by leadership. It creates a top-down filter of introspection and willingness to change. Once adopted, this culture becomes an integral part of the day-to-day operation of the entity.

While CQI catches mistakes and addresses issues in processes, the long-term result is overall improvements.

EXAMPLE OF AN INTERRELATED SYSTEM OF CARE

Let's apply a version of CQI and the 7 Cs in creating an inter-related system of care that will address the issues identified and include their value to stakeholders in the process. I've repeatedly demonstrated to colleagues that a solution exists for the myriad issues they identify in the service systems. When we dissect it, we truly become catalysts for change.

Figure 5.1 helps illustrate the simplest CQI model I could create. It is ideal because all three areas are adjacent to each other and cases can be easily moved from one to the other and back again. There's no restriction and no requirement to follow a defined pattern. You can create your own path on a case-by-case basis according to the needs of each individual. Only one rule applies: *On some level, you have to pay attention to all three areas.* At times, REVIEW will be most important; at times, PLAN will. Still other situations will rely heavily on DO. For example, you may walk into a case already at the REVIEW stage and determine it needs a better PLAN.

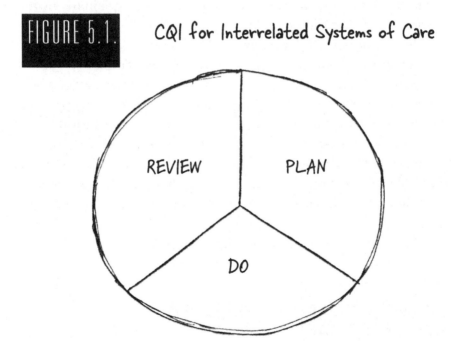

FIGURE 5.1. CQI for Interrelated Systems of Care

PLAN

Every day and repeatedly throughout the year, teams of key providers meet to design treatment plans for individuals in need of care. When discussing treatment, system representatives and providers begin with "discharge planning" if an individual is leaving a state or private facility, or "treatment planning" for those staying in the community.

Planning is the responsibility of local providers in consultation with clinical experts and countless others in both inpatient and outpatient settings. According to Medicare and the Joint Commission on the Accreditation of Healthcare Organizations (JCAHO), a plan should be reviewed every ninety days. This timeframe gives CQI a springboard for implementation.

None of this leads to suggesting that planning is easy. Given agency limitations, resource availability, client functioning, and client cooperation (or its lack), a realistic and attainable treatment plan is sometimes hard to pull off. But we need to start somewhere, and that's where the iterative process of CQI comes in. It allows us to revisit the plan, which we will look at later. But first we need to consider core elements of a plan's implementation.

Planning at all levels includes the individual client and his or her family. First, it's necessary to clearly identify the diagnoses and needs, as well as consider available services and those already being used. The planning process begins the moment an individual is hospitalized. If the individual lives in the community, planning needs to be continuous. Remember, a plan is iterative—a living, breathing, morphing concept. It's not stagnant and should never be considered permanent in any way.

I recently met with my twenty staff members to give them an example of how much their roles are appreciated and how much they need to value the work they do. None of them were with me at the time of Jeffrey's saga, so I wanted them to hear it. After I finished, I told them to think about what needed to happen to set Jeffrey and his team on the right track for appropriate treatment. This request was met with long pauses and silence in the room.

So I started them out with this: "As coordinators, the work you do is complex. Decisions you make every day about where to start and where to go next may be second nature to you now, but to many, they're overwhelming. I want you to appreciate and value all you do and what goes into it. This isn't a test. Simply think about what has to happen on both a broad scale and with the finer points. You all have the answers within you, and you'll all tackle this problem. But understand the process you go through in doing so. It's quite dynamic and impressive."

Similarly, here's what I'd like *you* to take away from this book. You've come to this profession as a calling. You create your own "call to action" several times a day as you use the tools demonstrated for you here. It's likely second nature for you. I'm merely asking you to draw resources from within and use the tools you already have in a structured and systematic manner. Then, you and other providers will be speaking a common language and using a common process. This is the ultimate Interrelated Service System.

On a personal level, if you take what's already inside and reflect on your skills related to the model I'm setting forth, you can fix the issues that are plaguing our dysfunctional systems of care. The Guardian Model is about being mindful and purposeful. Our achievements didn't happen by accident. Like the methods themselves, this program was created purposefully with a plan. It works.

Fifteen years after Jeffrey's case, I walked my team through the same process of thinking about the case and, together, we came up with a contemporary outline of the plan implemented for Jeffrey. Here's how the discussion went.

Someone suggested "the first thing we need to do is to get him out of jail and back to the hospital." That suggestion was the catalyst for a meaningful discussion in my office. Breaking it down, we developed the following simple questionnaire that would initiate all our inquiries. It became the guideline for the PLAN stage of our CQI and will serve as the beginning framework.

Action item: Have a similar discussion with your staff now. Go back and use these 7 Cs to create the first part of CQI: the PLAN.

PLAN QUESTIONNAIRE

Who needs to be there (aside from our client)?

Who should also be there?

Who should absolutely not be there?

What is the main focus/topic for discussion?

What are the proposals to address the topic?

Who is in the best position to meet the needs of each proposal?

What are barriers to meeting the proposals?

How can we collaboratively remove those barriers?

What does follow-up mean relative to this plan?

Who is responsible for follow-up?

DO

Now let's look at how we DO the plan. Of course, we should have taken a great deal of time to consider the 7 Cs when putting together our plan so a thorough review of the 7 Cs may be redundant.

Again, it's not the result as much as the process of getting there that teaches us how to use this model effectively. Learning to strategize hones our skills. Remember, we may be introduced to a case after someone has implemented a plan and even after it has been reviewed. So, acumen in using the 7 Cs is important throughout each stage. The PLAN, REVIEW, DO process is ongoing; it's not a one-time event. As stated earlier, it can start any place along the continuum.

The exercise of illustrating the use of the 7 Cs in each stage of Continuous Quality Improvement will serve to demonstrate the detail with which you do your job. This process will again cause you to think of the complex work you're doing, why you do it, and how you do it. Trust me, it's worth it, and you deserve it. The work you're doing is vitally important. You are changing lives, and it doesn't hurt to take a step back, acknowledge it, and give yourself a pat on the back now and again. Lord knows, no one is going to do it for you.

~

Jeffrey went back to the psychiatric unit in the hospital and was treated there for quite some time. However, he still had to face the music for the charges he had pending. The team held true to its representations, and the public defender's office brokered the appropriate deals to allow Jail Diversion to work closely with the prosecution and propose a plan that would keep Jeffrey out of jail for the charges he faced.

This brought about a complex set of circumstances worth discussing as we finish Jeffrey's story. It demonstrates how integral these 7 Cs are to the implementation of the PLAN—the DO part of CQI.

Because of his previous issues with the law, Jeffrey had gone through the court systems before. He'd been given many opportunities by different diversionary teams throughout various courts. As a minor, he'd used his "youthful offender" status. As an adult, he'd already gone through the criminal justice system's "Alternative to Incarceration" plan. He had also worked with the Jail Diversion folks through the mental health program to keep him out of incarceration.

Now he was returning to court to resolve the issues on his town green behavior and his outstanding warrants. While he was waiting for his case to be called, Jeffrey met Jen, a new Jail Diversion worker. Jen devised a plan for Jeffrey she'd used hundreds of times before with success in terms of securing release and dismissal of charges for similar clients.

Under her plan, Jeffrey would agree to regular check-ins with his mental health caseworker in the community. He would agree to take his medication, attend groups and a day program that would provide structure to his day, and he would avoid the use of drugs and alcohol.

These are unquestionably beneficial expectations for Jeffrey, and the court would be delighted to see his cooperation with this plan. The problem? This was the exact plan that had been used thirty minutes to the south in a different court by a different Jail Diversion specialist. The plan had failed and resulted in Jeffrey's commitment to the psychiatric unit from which he had eloped. It was a plan that would set up Jeffrey for failure.

Once again, the court sought to place the onus for Jeffrey's care squarely on Jeffrey's shoulders. This system allows those involved to simply sit back and heave a collective sigh of anguish when a client doesn't fulfill the most basic of expectations.

The system wasn't considering that Jeffrey was cognitively limited and impaired by his mental illness. He had no chance of living up to these expectations, which only served to frustrate the courts when he returned for another round of minor criminal infractions.

This is only one of many recurring failures of the system and not unique to Jeffrey. Sometimes people are so beset with mental illness and cognitive impairments that they cannot PLAN/DO/REVIEW for themselves.

Since the public defender's social worker was present in the meetings between Jen and Jeffrey, the "team" that originally met to secure his transfer out of jail was advised of the new/old plan being proffered. Naturally, this set off a chain of events to correct the recommendation to the court. The consistency of the presence of this particular social worker and the lack of consistency in the presence of the original Jail Diversion specialist illustrate this point as a whole.

The social worker reached out to me. I called Sara, my Care Coordinator, team members, and the former Jail Diversion specialist to communicate to them the proposal but also to get them to collaborate once again to affect the outcome we had proposed for Jeffrey.

Turning to the 7 Cs as her guide, Sara pulled and pushed the team into line according to the PLAN, giving each team member *including Jeffrey* a real opportunity to succeed. Let's look at how she did this in light of the new fact pattern.

CONSISTENT

The DO cycle of our model requires consistency when applying the plan. This is paramount so each team member and our mutual client understand what's expected and how/why other team members are counting on their piston to fire in the proverbial engine. Again, consistency means that all members will do their jobs as prescribed under the PLAN. It also means we would like to see services delivered in the same fashion by the same representatives when at all possible. However, consistency *does not* mean we should try to employ the same principles or practices time and time again when they've previously failed. Wasn't it Einstein who defined this as insanity?

Thankfully, we had consistency here in that the same public defender social worker could keep her eye on Jeffrey as he went through the criminal court process. When we have lack of consistency in this regard—that is, two different Jail Diversion folks working in two different locations—we end up with inefficiency and an ill-fated plan that had already been proven to fail.

COMMITTED

The team put the plan together in a thoughtful manner. To the team, it *was* realistic and attainable. Each team member had his or her assigned tasks under the plan and was committed to its implementation.

This reminds me of when I was in Little League. Plenty of times, I didn't want to leave a swimming pool to practice ball. My father insisted I go because I was a part of a team and my teammates counted on me to play my position. I had made a commitment and needed to see it through—a good lesson learned I still carry with me.

When we DO our PLAN, we need to know other team members are on board. We might assume that since they were part of creating the PLAN in the first place, they have a vested interest in seeing it through. But let's not be naïve. Many, many times I've sat in bigwig meetings with heads of state who shake hands and sing "kumbaya" only to leave the room and forget their promises to each other as if the meeting had never taken place.

We can be forgiving and say people "get busy." But we also know some folks simply don't follow through, some overpromise things they can't deliver, and some tell us anything we want to hear to get the meeting over with. This spirit of collaboration goes back to my Little League example. *We need to be able to count on each other.*

COLLABORATIVE

Jeffrey's team followed up on the PLAN created. The team members understood the importance of their individual roles and worked together to fulfill those roles and implement the plan. When they met barriers that could potentially jeopardize the PLAN, they collaborated in a way that allowed the success of Jail Diversion *and* provided Jeffrey with an opportunity to address his mental health needs in a setting other than incarceration.

As an aside, I'm confident that if this PLAN hadn't come together, Jeffrey would have spent countless months incarcerated. While there, he would have continued to act out due to his lack of control over mental illness.

COMMUNICATIVE

People need to continue to communicate, and when barriers arise, fellow team members can help brainstorm ways around them. When a part of the plan seems complete (or seems near impossible), this needs to be shared among the team so everyone can act accordingly. REVIEW starts to force its way into the process here. It necessarily becomes part of DO to ensure that issues and milestones are shared in "real time" among all PLAN participants.

Open communication keeps us moving forward proactively and alleviates issues that can arise when we react to acute moments of crisis in the DO stage of our cycle. This, in turn, minimizes the frequency of crises.

Having been involved in Jeffrey's case for a long time, I was available to him when he went through several different systems of care, including the criminal court process. I reviewed his plans throughout the years and was able to point out/communicate that it made little sense to apply the same diversionary tactics that had previously been attempted without success.

COMPREHENSIVE

Knowing we have a team of dedicated people is only half the battle. We want to be sure that the individuals represent their agencies comprehensively. It's vital that any resources that can be brought to bear on a given subject aren't held back.

Every tool available to us must be brought out so we can DO our PLAN efficiently. We don't need a hatchet to kill a mosquito, but it's nice to know one of our teammates has a hatchet. Here, team members used their respective positions to facilitate Jeffrey's move back to the appropriate treatment setting. They arranged for transportation and spoke to the appropriate people to ensure his plan would be implemented across disparate providers and offices, including the prosecution and the judge.

CLIENT-DRIVEN

Sara, our Care Coordinator, met with Jeffrey regularly and his team members and inpatient providers. They not only ascertained Jeffrey's wishes but also considered system limitations and offerings in light of his best interest and least restrictive means of intervention.

COORDINATED

Although it may seem unlikely in this particular matter, with so many players from different agencies and responsibilities, the coordination piece of Jeffrey's plan was not overly complicated. It was comprehensive in that we were initially focused on getting Jeffrey through the court process. The team members were well versed in their roles and used the power of their offices to accomplish the appropriate steps along the way.

But let's not overlook the vital role that coordination plays in monitoring and reporting. It was careful monitoring that caught the snafu with the diversionary plan, and reporting that alerted the rest of the team. Thereafter, the coordination piece assisted in facilitating communication between Jail Diversion offices to discern appropriate changes to their proposal.

While reading this section, did you think about the questions you needed to ask yourself? Refer to the DO Questionnaire on the next page for a few examples.

Jeffrey continues to be a challenge for the mental health system. He's in his thirties now, but he has little executive functioning and behaves like a young teenager. His case is quite unusual, especially in the way in which representatives from many different agencies and institutions came together with a likeminded focus on doing the best for a mutual client.

This is one case in one jurisdiction in one state. There's no reason the principles discussed here can't be replicated for thousands of individuals with mental illnesses, kids stuck in the child welfare system, or folks with developmental disabilities.

DO QUESTIONNAIRE

What part of the PLAN am I responsible
for implementing?

What parts of the PLAN need to happen before I can
do mine?

What parts of the PLAN depend upon completion
of mine?

Whom do I need to contact before I DO my part?

Whom do I need to contact *after* I DO my part?

Who should also be notified of my progress?

Who can help me to fulfill my obligations
under the PLAN?

What barriers might I face in implementing the PLAN?

What strategies can I use to overcome barriers?

REVIEW

The Care Coordinator provides the glue that holds the treatment team together. And the REVIEW step is when she earns her salt. The role is diverse and complex, and should touch on all aspects of the treatment plan and the team by using the tools in the toolbox—you guessed it, the 7 Cs.

During REVIEW, the Care Coordinator will be instrumental in identifying strengths and weaknesses of the PLAN as it zigzags through the DO stage.

At its core, the idea is to be proactive. More important than devising and implementing a PLAN is a *proactive* REVIEW of its successes and failures. Otherwise, we simply react to acute moments of crisis, which results in an inefficient and ineffective use of resources.

Think of it this way. You drive a car on four tires every day. Each tire is supposed to be inflated to 45 psi. If all the tires fit the bill except one, the car won't drive smoothly. If one tire is at 40 psi, you can live with it but you want to get the level back to where it functions best. If the psi plummets to 30 or 15 or 0, it jeopardizes the function of the entire car and can be dangerous. Further, inflating a tire from 35 to 45 psi is easy. Stop off at any gas station and you can still find air for free! But stabilizing an out-of-control automobile *isn't* so easy. You have to pull to the side of the road, empty the trunk, get out and set up the jack, lift the car, remove the tire, find the spare, and replace the bad one. Then you have to put it all back and repeat the process when you get the flat fixed! All that work, because you didn't take time to check the tire pressure periodically. Seems an inefficient use of time and resources, right?

Likewise, your team coordinator is responsible for periodically checking *(reviewing)* the "tire pressure" of your team members to be sure *all* are at 45 psi.

~

So, how are these 7 Cs applied here? The Care Coordinator will use them to address the following core principles to ensure the success of the PLAN.

Consistent: Are team members constantly and predictably applying their skills to the PLAN and the DO. Are there regular points of contact with the team members to ensure their agency is on board and actively participating?

Committed: Have all team members remained invested in the PLAN, and have they begun to apply their specific skillsets to their assigned tasks?

Collaborative: Are team members talking to each other regarding their roles under the PLAN, and is feedback positive and productive? Successful collaboration is met only when all parties to the PLAN understand their role and responsibility and don't feel they're unduly burdened or put upon under the DO aspect of the PLAN's implementation.

Communicative: Is the coordinator able to reach necessary parties and get timely responses from them relative to the PLAN?

Comprehensive: When team members are applying their skills to the PLAN, are they using all the resources at their disposal?

Client-driven: Regular check-ins with the mutual client are absolutely necessary to ensure this most important cog in the wheel is still on board, seeing benefits, and actively participating to the extent possible.

Every time we walk up to our car, we look at our tires. We do this semiconsciously, and if we don't check the opposite side, most cars these days will tell us if one of the tires is flat. The point is that we have a mechanism in place to constantly check the baseline level of the function of our tires. By not allowing our clients to "crash," they see benefit to the PLAN and are willing to engage in it further.

Coordinated: When all the other Cs are in place, the plan is considered well-coordinated. If the other Cs are not in place, the Care Coordinator needs to pull the various players back together to make them aware of the unresolved issues and have them revisit the planning stage if necessary.

REVIEW OUTCOMES

In short, Care Coordinators are responsible for ensuring that when team members DO the PLAN, the following outcomes are achieved:

- *Expectation that change is possible.*

- *Movement away from acceptance of the status quo and a refocus on what can be done as opposed to what the team is prevented from doing.*

- *Proactive approach to treatment/recovery, starting from the administrative level and demonstrated to the staff in all agencies.*

- *Sense of understanding the limitations of clients and systems.*

- *Acceptance and expectation of setbacks. After all, this is the entire point of the REVIEW stage of this process.*

- *Empowerment of our mutual client in planning beyond a one-service system.*

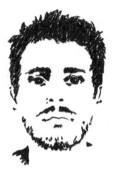

JAKE'S STORY

This situation is an example of when DOing the PLAN fell apart when the REVIEW stage was missing.

Jake has been living in an apartment his father built for him by converting the ground floor of their rural ranch-style home. His comprehensive team of providers works to "wrap him up" with services. The goal is to ensure he has a reasonable chance of remaining in the community he's known his whole life.

Jake is fiercely independent. However, he still relies on his father to maintain housing, transportation, and occasional meals. This is true of many clients who adamantly oppose intervention while feeling entitled to what keep them relatively safe in the community.

Another truth is that Jake's father has a life of his own! Every Autumn when the geese head south for the winter, Jake's dad follows them. It's his way of maintaining a degree of happiness and fulfillment for himself and his wife. Good for him!

In the fall, it becomes more important than ever that Jake's team rally to predict his needs over the coming months *and* create a plan to address any crises that may occur. The Care Coordinator is responsible for making sure these meetings occur. Jake is always a challenge, and these months make him even more so, given the absence of his father who can't check in and report his well-being to the Care Coordinator. (Note: Jake's father is an integral part of the RE-VIEW process.) So they created a plan in which the case management team from the local mental health provider would be responsible for wellness checks on Jake on a "regular" basis.

A word of caution: Terms such as "regular" are dangerous in the PLAN stage. They're defined differently during the DO stage when the reality of busy schedules often gets in the way. In Jake's case, "regular" changed from weekly to monthly and disintegrated from there. So in planning, it's to everyone's benefit for these terms to be clearly defined.

During one wellness check at the apartment, the case manager was greeted by an ornery Jake, who told her to go away in vulgar terms. He even slammed the door on her! The process was repeated the next week and the week after that. The Care Coordinator in this case was frantic. No one had actually laid eyes on Jake in a month. The primary care provider (PCP) and clinical team were concerned about his adhering to his medication regimen. The coordinator's efforts to persuade the case managers to be more creative in their engagement techniques fell on deaf ears. Likewise, the case management supervisors took an adversarial approach to the coordinator and advised her they were working under a "recovery-oriented system of care" and that "client choice must be honored above all else."

> *I call this the stupidity defense. In its "logical"*
> *application, it says that individuals have the*
> *right to make bad decisions even if 1) they are*
> *cognitively incapable of understanding the dire*
> *ramifications of the decision, and/or 2) they*
> *don't have the mental capacity to make any*
> *decisions given the degree of their illness. Under*

*this argument, people's rights to make bad
decisions should be protected, even if doing so
may result in harm to themselves or others.*

*Does this mean we should allow people to
die with their boots and their rights on?*

Jake was a conserved individual who was legally declared to be incapable of making informed decisions about his health care. His fiduciary was mandated to ensure his safety and shelter and that his daily needs were met. Providers had agreed on a treatment plan that included outreach to Jake, who had no means of obtaining food other than through his providers. Arguably, the providers are mandated reporters and had a duty to ensure Jake's health and safety.

However, Jake was difficult, impolite, and downright rude to them, so the decision to stop engagement was probably an easy one. Two weeks later, however, Jake was rushed to the hospital with advanced liver failure and other life-threatening illnesses. He hadn't eaten or had anything to drink during the time this debacle was unfolding!

An advocate for Jake was quoted as saying, "Even my dog knows enough to drink when he's thirsty." This wasn't an attempt at dark humor. Rather, it's social commentary on the fact that it's easy to hide behind what's perceived to be the "rights" of individuals to protect their dignity. Meanwhile, there's no dignity in the endgame of liver and kidney dysfunction. We wouldn't let a dog suffer this way, and it seems criminal to allow a human being to do so in the name of "client choice."

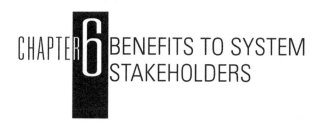

CHAPTER 6 BENEFITS TO SYSTEM STAKEHOLDERS

Frankly, when I set out to create The Guardian Model, I didn't anticipate the breadth of its impact. I was the unwelcome coordinator that others perceived as a threat, a watchdog, a bully, or a babysitter. But as with anything worth doing, the growing pains reap their rewards, and I can honestly say that systems embracing the concepts delineated here have benefited tremendously from the program.

Statistically speaking, we're on course to save millions of dollars for our stakeholders this year. After the initial discomfort of "sibling rivalry," providers have welcomed us as an integral member of the team, and together we show reductions in recidivism to hospitals and emergency rooms, arrests, and incarcerations. Episodes of prolonged institutionalization have decreased, along with the number of days per stay. Individuals claim an increased sense of involvement in treatment and a higher life satisfaction overall.

I didn't anticipate the value that so many different stakeholders would see in programs such as this. I'm proud that these concepts, simple in design but tough in application, have benefited so many people, families, loved ones, and organizations. The impact goes far beyond the number of clients directly served. Results are being realized exponentially across the entire spectrum of care and, for that reason, aren't easily quantifiable.

I'm most impressed with and touched by family members who thank us for changing their lives by changing the lives of their loved ones. We're empowering individuals to take an active part in planning for their future. The quality of life spreads like laughter across social and political boundaries, between silos of corporate and institutional isolation, and through the doors of resentment and anger that often impede healthy, interpersonal relationships.

Consider these examples.

FAMILY MEMBERS/FIDUCIARY

Through this program, family members and/or fiduciaries of persons in need are afforded an ally who can assist them in understanding the intricacies of the myriad systems in which the individual is involved. They're given a better understanding of the complexities of each particular case, a sounding board for their frustrations, and an effective voice for relating their position as it pertains to their loved one or client.

Additionally, the program alleviates micromanagement of daily needs. Family members can go on with their own lives knowing a responsive, caring group is watching over their loved one and assuring his/her needs are met.

The fiduciary is also relieved on many levels, which differ in some instances. By receiving regular contact and reports as required by The Model, the fiduciary can feel at ease, knowing that individuals are receiving the services they are entitled to, and feel that they are safe in the community.

PROBATE COURT

By providing a service to the fiduciary, The Model serves as an invaluable component of the courts' overall ability to serve persons in need. The attorneys who frequently practice in these courts know their fiduciary responsibilities will be less burdensome with this level of assistance. Thus, the number of those willing to participate increases.

When courts have access to a larger pool of responsible and qualified individuals willing to serve, its efficiency in hearing these matters and moving them forward to a positive resolution increases. Likewise, through oversight, The Model has demonstrated that the court is less likely to be burdened with people in need who frequently pass through its revolving doors on their way to successive processes.

LOCAL MENTAL HEALTH AUTHORITY

I initially anticipated that the Local Mental Health Authority (LMHA) working with persons who have mental illnesses would present the most resistance to The Model. This, however, has proven to be far from true. Caseworkers see The Model as a valuable ally with access to administrative personnel who otherwise may not get involved in particular cases. In this manner, the team can move past typical bureaucratic roadblocks to affect positive change for the client's benefit.

LMHA caseworkers have noted that The Model is an integral piece in facilitating open lines of communication between themselves, their subcontracted service providers, and the fiduciary caring for a client. They can obtain documentation in a timely manner, as well as vital information regarding the individual. Records on treatment history, successes, and failures are diligently maintained and disseminated.

HOSPITALS

In addition to providing an accessible representative who can facilitate communication that's never before been available to hospital staff and personnel, The Model is a source of vital information. The Guardian Model follows a client across all agencies and through all systems in the community. Thus, it can provide the hospital with documented evidence of a client's treatment history, medications, compliance, and overall condition in the community. The Model makes available to all providers a comprehensive picture of the circumstances that affect a client's care.

Intimate knowledge of the client, including his/her needs and successes in the community, makes The Model a link to the community and an asset to the development of new, comprehensive, and realistic discharge plans.

DEPARTMENT OF MENTAL HEALTH (DMH)

Unfortunately, financial considerations are a part of today's world. Resources are carefully distributed among various service agencies, which do everything possible to work within tight, inflexible budgets. The Model has proven to be a valuable asset to the DMH. There, the number of man-hours previously needed to treat the most "difficult" clients is greatly reduced. Providers often become disinclined to treat the chronically mentally ill as prescribed by their treatment plan and under their contract with the Department. That's due to factors such as burnout, lack of engagement, lack of client commitment, or simply frustration of not moving the ball forward. Through collaboration and accountability, this responsibility for action among subcontracted service agencies is distributed appropriately.

By reducing the number of bed days in private as well as state hospitals, the Department has saved money that can be reallocated to benefit other clients in need and/or develop programs to reduce the overutilization of services.

In many cases, input of other agencies and departments is sought in developing courses of treatment and obtaining needed services across the fictitious boundaries. That means outside agencies, better suited for addressing particular needs of a client, assume some of (if not all) the costs of delivering the most appropriate responses. Again, this frees assets and manpower to effectively address the services the Department could and should be asked to handle.

CRIMINAL JUSTICE SYSTEM

The Department of Corrections (DOC) and the criminal justice continuum are necessary components of the mental health system. However, they're being misused. This is primarily due to a lack of understanding of what the mentally ill need and the chronic nature of mental illness itself. Added to that is a failure to distinguish criminality from the manifestation of an illness.

Many detainees with a history of mental illness shouldn't be in jail. They won't benefit from—indeed, they can't understand—the causal link between their actions and their punishment, such as incarceration. DOC spends tens of thousands of dollars to treat their prisoners with drugs. When people are discharged, they aren't given a comprehensive plan. Homelessness becomes pervasive, leading to criminal behavior, which lands the client back within the criminal justice system.

By avoiding incarceration, we avoid taxing the criminal justice system. By acting as an information resource, The Model influences the efficiency of the criminal justice system and its ability to handle this unique population. As a result, incarceration is no longer the only answer to chronic offenders who have mental health issues.

Anywhere the client may fall within the criminal justice/mental health continuum can benefit from the consistency and knowledge The Guardian Model offers. The Model can assist police in understanding the client's behaviors prior to or directly after detention. It can assist Jail Diversion or Alternative to Incarceration programs in developing strategies that may never have been tried and avoid duplicating those that have previously failed. It can assure courts that a thoughtful review of each person's case and circumstances leading to arrest can assist in identifying criminality versus illness. It acts as the ongoing provider to the client, following that person's progress through all aspects of community life. The result is a decrease in recidivism or a better understanding of why it may happen.

It doesn't take much to understand this program's expansive reach to people involved in the lives of each individual participant. Can you think of others that would benefit from this type of collaboration? There are likely many!

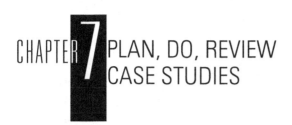
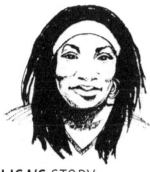

LISA'S STORY

Lisa is a forty-five-year-old black woman who's had moderate success living in the community. However, she has a diagnosis of paranoid schizophrenia, which seriously affects her ability to maintain stability in the community and get treatment for end-stage renal failure.

She uses the hospital emergency room for her primary care *and* as a means to manipulate staff at the assisted living facility where she resides. Lisa is convinced that case managers are conspiring against her and that every male in the facility wants to rape her or kill her or both. She has an uncanny ability to induce in herself a catatonic state. Then she shuts down for long periods and cannot or will not be brought back to lucidity.

Her renal failure demands that she receive dialysis for several hours three days a week. However, due to

her paranoia, Lisa becomes disruptive and combative with pa-
trons and staff in a clinical setting. She doesn't want to undergo
dialysis and no one is willing to assist her. The specialist who treats
Lisa for her renal disease believes that, if Lisa is inconsistent with
her dialysis treatment, it can be just as dangerous as if she's not
receiving treatment at all. Given her inclination to decline treatment and her paranoia, he and Lisa have decided the best course
of action for her is to avoid dialysis altogether.

When she was admitted to a large teaching hospital, it forced
the ethics of Lisa's case to be discussed. The leading nephrologist
on staff felt strongly that he could and should treat Lisa's renal
failure appropriately. Community providers cautioned she would
be unlikely to remain consistent once she was released from the
hospital. The medical unit was having difficulty managing Lisa's
behavior. The staff wanted to move her to a psychiatric floor.
However, members of the psychiatric unit staff claimed they were
incapable of managing Lisa's medical needs.

A review of her medical history indicated that Lisa functioned
at or near her "base line" for the longest period when she was given
lithium. Yet lithium and other psychotropic medications are processed through the liver and can be damaging to it. Lisa couldn't
afford to have liver damage. However, with no medication, her behavior was difficult to manage—and thus the dilemma.

Wanting to be discharged to a nearby city, Lisa refused to continue working with her current treatment providers. She declared
she would live in the home of an elderly cousin she hadn't spoken
to in twenty years. Her father and mother were despondent over
this. They desperately wanted Lisa to receive dialysis to give her
a chance at survival. They were able to reach her better than
most people and believed that, if given an opportunity, they could
influence her psychosis treatment. To date, however, her parents
had not been invited to the "table" to assist.

Her parents hoped Lisa could maintain a meaningful life in the
community. But where could she live? The idea of placing her in
a nursing home was uncomfortable given her relatively young age.

However, it did offer the best "control" setting to treat her dialysis. Having an independent apartment with wraparound supports was considered, but most of the team didn't think she had the life skills to live on her own, and she'd be inclined to miss dialysis.

Further, although she was extremely thin, Lisa was a huge fan of any kind of junk food and would gorge herself at every opportunity. This, too, threatened her kidney function. Current rooming houses, group homes, and other congregate settings wouldn't consider welcoming Lisa, given both her long history of noncompliance and the complications associated with her medical needs.

The team needed a plan. It had nothing in place for Lisa, particularly given her steadfast refusal to continue to work with her case management provider. She wasn't welcome back to her apartment and ran the risk of losing her housing voucher if her landlord pursued a summary process eviction as he had threatened. The community medical personnel were at odds with the inpatient staff. Meanwhile, Lisa's underlying psychosis was going untreated and spiraling steadily downward.

At this stage, I was appointed as conservator/guardian of Lisa, and I walked right into the hornet's nest. My team and I deliberated over this case and used the tools shared in this book to guide the entire treatment team. Because there was no viable scheme in place, we started with our own plan.

PLAN QUESTIONNAIRE

Who needs to be there (aside from our client)?

Lisa was incapable of participating in treatment planning at this stage. She was floridly psychotic and refused to talk to anyone except her nephrologist, whom she felt was in love with her. Therefore, I had to act as a surrogate decision maker for Lisa, and I started with her health issues. I learned her nephrologist was convinced of two things: 1) She should be treated for her renal failure or she would certainly die, and 2) she should be treated again with lithium to enable her to maintain a baseline level of control.

Unsure, I coordinated several discussions among her community physician, the lead inpatient nephrologist, and me. Our ongoing concern was that Lisa would be discharged and wouldn't have any place to receive dialysis if she did want to go.

Who should also be there?

The Department of Mental Health played an important role when representatives joined our meetings and had their utility management team "fast-track" a placement for Lisa at the only remaining state operated psychiatric hospital. This was no small feat because 1) the hospital was the subject of a Department of Justice oversight plan regarding the discharge of patients, and 2) the hospital already had a long wait list for admissions.

But the hospital could do what no place else was capable of doing. *It could address Lisa's underlying psychiatric needs and provide her with dialysis on-site.* It was absolutely the only option. Not a long-term fix but at least it provided a step in the right direction. Lisa was "prioritized" and admitted.

Who should absolutely not be there?

Given Lisa's attitude toward her community treatment providers, I felt uneasy about including them in meetings to discuss planning. However, they had worked with her for years and, along with her parents, were the best source of information to assist in discharge and treatment planning.

Likewise, I reasoned that Lisa's angst with them was quite likely born from her paranoia as opposed to any legitimate differences, as was her reported perception. This would later prove to be a lesson learned repeatedly throughout my career. As irrational as people may seem at any given time, no matter how delusional or paranoid they are, it's important to remember *this is their reality.* We have to start our work from this point and, figuratively, meet them where they are. Given the many, many layers of this particular onion, I wanted as many hands and hearts and minds at the table as possible. My approach is to connect the experts and follow their advice when at all possible.

In the spirit of engagement and empowerment, therefore, it's important that, at least initially, we don't include in meetings with our mutual client people who may be perceived as a threat or "malevolent" in the client's mind. This could be a family member, a particular clinician or caseworker, a hospital/court representative, or even a fiduciary. The initial planning and meeting stage will set the tenor for what follows and can lay a critical foundation for the work we do moving forward.

What is the main focus/topic for discussion?

Clearly, the main topic for discussion was the immediate need for placement and treatment of Lisa. But a slew of subtopics needed to be addressed as well. For instance, should we give her dialysis treatment despite the advice of her community physician and against her wishes? How would this even work? Given her age and her proclivity toward disruptive behavior, how viable would nursing home placement be? What community setting would be best for her and where would she be physically located?

What are the proposals to address the topic?

Because Lisa needed to stabilize, the inpatient nephrologist proposed her taking lithium again at a lower dosage than before.

Who is in the best position to meet the needs of each proposal?

The nephrologist prescribed a dosage of lithium to be given to Lisa at night *after* she had undergone dialysis (so the process wouldn't flush the drug out of her system).

Her parents had a long, heartfelt meeting with Lisa and convinced her that they loved her. They wanted more than anything for her to survive and overcome her challenges—and this meant dialysis.

What are barriers to meeting the proposals?

Ethics and the damage lithium could do to Lisa's condition were a major concern. Also of concern was her absolute refusal to continue with dialysis and her relationship with her community-based case management team.

How can we collaboratively remove those barriers?

Conversations between physicians proved fruitful and positive despite their differences of opinion. Ultimately, however, the in-patient nephrologist felt an obligation to use all of his resources to treat Lisa. He and I discussed my fear that Lisa would be prematurely discharged with no follow-up plan and only a halfhearted effort to address her medical needs once she began to show the slightest signs of lucidity.

What does follow-up mean relative to this plan?

The first phase in this plan was to achieve psychiatric stability and implement dialysis. Once we had those two factors down, we could plan again for a second phase of Lisa's treatment.

Who is responsible for follow-up?

Given my fiduciary role and the fact that I run a nonprofit agency for this purpose, I was the likely candidate to ensure this stage of the PLAN was implemented and successful. I'm happy to say Lisa did clear up slightly, began dialysis, and was moved to the state psychiatric hospital. There, we continued to treat her according to the PLAN set forth until it became feasible for her to move to a more permanent setting.

In this case, the PLAN was not overly complicated but arriving at a consensus was. Likewise, once the PLAN was agreed upon, the DO and REVIEW stages were highly dictated by Lisa's psychiatric and medical treatment needs. Permanent placement and ongoing treatment would be the next set of challenges for us. The most obvious barriers were availability of housing and Lisa's strong opinions about what she wanted and where she would live. The Guardian Model gives the team step-by-step instructions to follow to tackle each consecutive challenge.

While Lisa was an inpatient, an Occupational Therapy (OT) assessment indicated a need for 24-hour support including prompting, assistance with activities of daily living (ADL) needs, and otherwise managing her care. Lisa also had to reside in a place with female peers due to her trauma history and ongoing delusions around males.

At the time, several of our clients were being placed in newly designed "permanent" homes. One was a home for women with acute psychiatric disorders, and with the help of the medical director of the Department of Mental Health, Lisa was sent there. A further assessment was performed, and from there, Lisa was linked with a new community provider and a dialysis center to treat her on an outpatient basis.

This PLAN sounds straightforward and relatively successful. However, Lisa's behavior continues to be problematic in a community setting. She frequently uses trips to the hospital as a maladaptive coping mechanism, and she accuses staff and male peers of inappropriate behaviors. As I was writing this, a coordinator on my staff came into my office to advise me that Lisa was being brought to the hospital. She was seriously decompensating while exhibiting manifestations of her mental illness as well as her recently identified behavioral disorders.

As a community provider working with Lisa, what would you do to ensure she's given the proper tools to live in the community? What types of training would you and your peers need to work with Lisa? Picture yourself as her clinician or her case manager. Perhaps you are the director of the residential facility. How can you continue to keep Lisa in the community, given the multitude of issues she presents? Remember, she needs dialysis, psychotropic medication, and a behavioral plan. How would you address these questions?

This is where you DO the PLAN.

DO QUESTIONNAIRE

What part of the PLAN am I responsible for implementing?

What parts of the PLAN need to happen before I can do mine?

What parts of the PLAN depend upon completion of mine?

Whom do I need to contact before I DO my part?

Whom do I need to contact *after* I DO my part?

Who should also be notified of my progress?

Who can help me to fulfill my obligations under the PLAN?

What barriers might I face in implementing the PLAN?

What strategies can I use to overcome barriers?

REVIEW QUESTIONNAIRE

Given Lisa's ongoing use of the hospital, I get frequent calls advising me of her status. This isn't all that helpful because these calls are little more than the admissions office at a metropolitan hospital calling me for permission to treat. One of my greatest difficulties is navigating the telephone system at the hospital to get to the right party who can tell me her status. Therefore, I rely heavily on a wonderful care coordinator, Jaimie, in my office who monitors and reports on Lisa to me. I ask Jaimie to share details of her role and how the REVIEW part of a case proceeds on a daily basis.

Here's the e-mail I sent to my team: *Each caseworker is assigned a specific caseload and they stick to that caseload along with their supervisor, clinical director, and support staff.*

You'll recognize the questions I posit are based around the 7 Cs in a manner my team understands. This shows our dialogue and how we regularly communicate. I encourage you to adapt these lines of questioning and verbiage in your thinking as well:

To: All Staff
CC:
Subject: Lisa
From: Michael Mackniak

Okay, what I need from you guys is a detailed account of what you do to monitor Lisa's case. (REVIEW COORDINATED)

Who are you talking to? (COMMUNICATE, COLLABORATE)

Is the team following the plan? (COMMITTED)

Is the team communicating and collaborating?

Is Lisa involved or even capable of being involved? (CLIENT-DRIVEN)

Does the approach to treatment follow the PLAN?

Are individual providers regularly involved? (CONSISTENT)

Are we using all resources at our disposal?

Is there a behavioral plan?

Is there more we can or should be doing? (COMPREHENSIVE)

And here was the response:

To: Michael Mackniak
CC:
Subject: Lisa
From: Sara

There is weekly communication with Residential, Mental Health, Nursing, and Case Management. There are weekly meetings at Mental Health with Residential to problem solve and follow up on recommendations.

Case Management has gone out to Lotus House to do diet teaching. They send monthly reports on how she is doing with recommendations, which are then sent to Residential and disseminated to the team by us. Lisa has also received the training on her diet and has been involved with the process of her diet choices. Interventions were put in place for cheat days, fluid restrictions, etc. She also goes to dialysis with snacks and something to do to keep her distracted. At times, items were forgotten, but the team communicates when this happens and reminders are noted for staff at Residential. Extra staff has been added at times when dialysis is increased due to an increase of fluid retention.

ER visits, when she was first using the ER, we assessed that it was due to her blood pressure. The team advocated for an appointment, medications were adjusted, and issues resolved. Then the ER visits were for falls in the home, mostly around stairs. An OT evaluation was completed and safety in the house was addressed. After this, the ER visits appeared to be attention-seeking behaviors. Currently, the team has talked about getting a behavioral consultant to create a behavioral plan that would help decrease the number of ER visits. The team could also explore appropriate treatment and provide recommendations, such as CBT, DBT, or trauma therapy.

The psychiatrist reviewed medications and is making adjustments with her Haldol. Medication history was provided from records collected from past hospitalizations and consultations with DMH and Psych hospital. There will always need to be a balance due to renal failure and sensitivity to medications that could be beneficial psychiatrically.

What needs to be further explored are her family members. They've been more involved in the past and have been helpful with treatment and encouragement. The other thing is trying to find something she wants to do so she's not at the house all day—maybe work or volunteering somewhere.

Something else that's being explored is the Behavioral Health Home (BHH) or Intensive Case Management to offer intensive case management for the ER visits. The case managers could go to the ER when Lisa arrives and help coordinate psych and mental health care for her and the team. They could connect her with a PCP she may use and assist with other medical education around her dialysis.

I also speak with the conservator of the estate regularly. Many of the incentives around following through with medical tasks are financial and involve additional expenditure of money or receiving money sooner so she can go shopping.

VIGNETTES

Your toolbox is full. You've seen how these 7 Cs are constructed and how they combine for the Big C, which is Continuous Quality Improvement. You can now determine if you and your agency are ready to use these tools across your system of care.

Next, you'll read more examples of real cases and you're encouraged to pick them apart. Most of these scenarios will sound familiar to you on one level or another. At first, you'll find cases illustrating questions that apply to each of the 7 Cs. They're noted for you, when and where you need to recognize their impact. Look for illustrations of problems with the Big C, either in the PLAN, DO, or REVIEW stage.

Finally, take the initiative to dissect fact patterns and practice the skills you've developed so far. There's no right or wrong answer; the action of going through the exercise is equally as important as the result you aim to achieve. This is particularly true considering that, ultimately, the continuous quality improvement diagram is designed so you can recheck your work in the spirit of constructive criticism and proactively addressing shortcomings.

Pretend you're starting from scratch. Do you need a PLAN? Is a PLAN in place that's not working and needs to be REVIEWED first? Then revisit the questionnaires provided. Use them in concert with the 7 Cs as you work through creating realistic and attainable goals for your client and the entire team of providers.

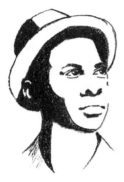

WALLACE'S STORY

Wallace is a twenty-seven-year-old African American male diagnosed with schizoaffective disorder, cocaine dependence, PTSD, ADHD (by history), and antisocial personality disorder. Since childhood, he's had a long history of mental illness, trauma, and involvement with the law.

He was residing in the community with his aunt in her apartment, assigned to ACT (ASSERTIVE COMMUNITY TREATMENT TEAM) level of services, and on probation. (COLLABORATION AND COMMUNICATION)

Wallace was a challenge to engage, often frequented the local ERs, actively used substances, and was noncompliant with medications, treatment, and his legal issues. (COORDINATED)

He spent a lot of time wandering the streets, which concerned his providers as he consistently put himself at risk for unsafe situations, e.g., getting loud with others, walking into traffic, and so on.

His team had struggled to engage him. They had made appointments to meet with him in the home and sought him out in his neighborhood and known hangouts, but they were never able to connect with him. (COMMITTED)

They'd tried behavioral contracts and rewards, and had attempted to educate him on the possible consequences of his behaviors and noncompliance, to no avail. (COMPREHENSIVE)

The team's plan was for risk reduction, to do as much as Wallace would allow them to do, and to attempt to get him to engage. (CLIENT-DRIVEN)

They needed to identify the barriers and different possible strategies to try. (COLLABORATIVE)

It was discovered that Wallace would stay out late and his aunt would lock the doors after a certain hour so that after that time Wallace didn't have access to the home. This would often lead him into the ER, where he would have shelter for the night. In the early morning, he'd report that he was feeling better and be discharged home, at which time he had access to enter. (COMMUNICATIVE, CONSISTENT)

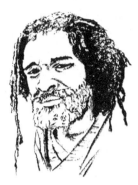

JACK'S STORY

Jack is a fifty-six-year-old African American male diagnosed with schizophrenia, polysubstance dependence (full remission), and mild developmental disability (WAIS-R Full Scale IQ of 45, Verbal IQ of 55).

Jack has an extensive history of hospitalizations and legal issues. In addition, he's an extremely high user of emergency rooms in and outside the region. This has become a major concern for community providers and the hospitals themselves. (COLLABORATIVE AND COMMUNICATIVE)

The client was residing in his own apartment with Department of Developmental Disabilities (DDS) supports in place while receiving outpatient mental health treatment from the local mental health authority. (COMPREHENSIVE) He struggled in this environment, so it was determined he required more intensive supports.

As a high user of the ER, Jack was also an identified client for the community care team. Multiple people involved in his care, from both the community and the hospitals, committed to gather to identify strategies of how to work collaboratively in decreasing ER visits. (COMMITTED, COMPREHENSIVE)

Unfortunately, even with these combined efforts, his daily visits to the ER continued. (COORDINATED, CONSISTENT) His underlying reasons for going to the ER (despite his reports of presenting concerns) were actually related to his perception that the ER would provide him with additional bus tokens or food he liked. (CLIENT-DRIVEN)

The client often presented to the ER saying he had no medications, so the ER would provide his meds. This became a significant risk factor because one entity was not aware of what was happening with other entities. Consequently, the client was receiving double doses of his medications on a regular basis. (COMMUNICATIVE AND COLLABORATIVE)

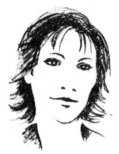

KELLIE

Kellie was homeless and on the street. She had been diagnosed with bipolar disorder and her last test results showed she had an IQ under 60. She'd been through four apartments in the last two years. Each time, people from the community would start to live there, and on one occasion, people took her key and refused to allow her to stay. Years of cocaine use and prostitution had taken their toll on Kellie. Her self-esteem was depleted, and she had no hope for change.

Finally, it was decided a supervised apartment might be the right level of care. Three agencies looked at Kellie's referral, and they were sure she wouldn't do well in their programs. She had been sexually assaulted the week before and someone had to give her the chance she needed.

PLAN: KELLIE

How do we break the cycle of drug abuse and prostitution?

Can Kellie understand/benefit from an inpatient substance-abuse setting?

How can we convince a residential provider to take her into their program?

What can we offer the provider in additional support & training?

Who needs to be there (aside from our client)?

Who should also be there?

Who should absolutely not be there?

What is the main focus/topic for discussion?

What are the proposals to address the topic?

Who is in the best position to meet the needs of each proposal?

What are barriers to meeting the proposals?

How can we collaboratively remove those barriers?

What does follow-up mean relative to this plan?

Who is responsible for follow-up?

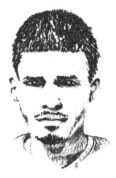

CONNOR

Connor had spent three years in a state hospital. The discharge plan was ready. He would go back to the area he was from and live in a group home geared to working with people who had addictions. He would go to groups and be expected to abstain from using his drug of choice, cocaine. The first week of discharge went well, but shortly after that, calls started coming in from providers.

Connor was not doing well. He was urinating in jars again in his room. He was not coming home on time. He was not attending groups, and he was using drugs again. Connor was also missing medications, which was never a good sign.

Numerous meetings and interventions were held, but something was missing. After a year of failed interventions, the team explored other possible options: Would Connor do better in a program that had more structure? Would he do better in a program geared toward working on helping him with his symptoms in addition to his addiction? Would he attend the groups associated with a structured group home?

DO: CONNOR

Who is the prescribed intervener for Connor when he begins to refuse medication?

What incentive have we provided to get Connor to maintain medication compliance?

Who is to address the unprovoked manner of Connor's outbursts?

Who is reviewing the medications that Connor is supposed to take in order to determine their efficacy?

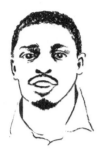

RYAN

Ryan had only lived in the community for six months of the last three years. He had a troubled past and carried a diagnosis of schizophrenia. He used cannabis and cocaine to self-medicate, as he felt more in control when he used.

Ryan was happy on most days, but he struggled with the symptoms associated with his illness. He experienced auditory hallucinations that would at times "trick" him. He would often think people were talking about him, and on several occasions he became physically violent.

During the last incident, he pushed a staff person into a plate-glass window after assaulting a peer. The incident was unprovoked.

Ryan would be admitted to the hospital, stay for a couple of months, and then get discharged into a supervised apartment program. He'd then stop taking medications, start abusing substances, and assault someone. He was trapped in the revolving door of recidivism.

REVIEW: RYAN

What interventions do we need to implement in order to DO the
PLAN more effectively?

Is this the right level of care?

Have we addressed psychosis and drug dependence?

Can he participate in groups and other requirements of congregate living settings?

Did our plan implement these 7 Cs?

- *Consistent*
- *Committed*
- *Collaborative*
- *Communicative*
- *Comprehensive*
- *Client-driven*
- *Coordinated*

GENERAL CASE STUDIES: YOUR TURN

In reviewing these cases, first figure out which stage of the Big C we're at. Should we be at this stage, or do we need to move forward or backward to address the problems faced in each scenario? Then we need to get an understanding of the individual needs of each case. How are they unique? How are they similar? Have we seen this before? What's the most important aspect of each to tackle? Prioritize!

Use the questions. The answers are in the 7 Cs. Apply them to each.

Don't underestimate the impact you can have, both in your organization and in your clients' lives.

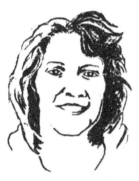

MARY

Mary is a fifty-eight-year-old white single female with a diagnosis of schizoaffective disorder, borderline personality disorder, and multiple medical diagnoses such as diabetes. She has a long history of residing in a nursing home level of care. The nursing home was closed and Mary was moved to a rest home, where she resided for a year and then transitioned to her own apartment.

She began to have an increase in mental health symptoms and was admitted to a local hospital. The team met to discuss level of care options and decided to try another rest home and then a Department of Mental Health group home. Both were unsuccessful, and she was admitted to a long-term bed at a state-run psych facility. Mary reported to the team that she wanted her own apartment with support.

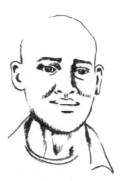

CHARLIE

Charlie is a fifty-five-year-old single African American male with a diagnosis of schizophrenia and opioid dependence. He had a long history of hospitalizations, incarcerations, and homelessness. Charlie struggles with heroin and alcohol abuse.

He was residing in a rooming house, using substances, and not taking prescribed psychiatric medications. The team got together to discuss how best to work with Charlie. Treatment was recommended, but Charlie refused.

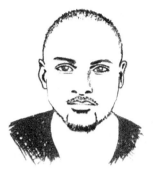

TODD

Todd is a forty-two-year-old single African-American male with a diagnosis of schizoaffective disorder, cannabis abuse, and antisocial personality disorder. He had an intensive history of hospitalizations and incarcerations starting in the 1980s. He has paranoid thoughts and delusions. He often reports being able to raise and set the sun, caring for his multiple children that he doesn't have, and seeing the boogieman outside of his apartment. Todd was admitted to the state psychiatric hospital after legal involvement, assaults, and breach of peace. He couldn't reside in congregate housing as he had numerous interpersonal conflicts with peers.

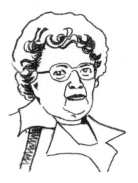

JEN

Jen is a seventy-four-year-old divorced Caucasian woman with a diagnosis of schizoaffective disorder. She was moved to an apartment due to affordability, but she isn't familiar with the area and her new surroundings. She struggles with interpersonal relationships, especially with those who reside around her due to her paranoid and delusional thought processes.

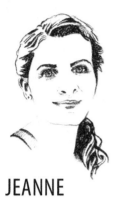

JEANNE

Jeanne is a forty-year-old single Caucasian woman with a diagnosis of depressive disorder, alcohol abuse, pyromania, and neurodevelopmental disorder. She was incarcerated at York Correctional Facility after setting the trailer of a man she was interested in on fire while under the influence of alcohol.

Family had contacted the agency for assistance after stating feelings of frustration with the lack of services available for their daughter.

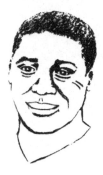

MARK

Mark is a forty-five-year-old single African-American male with a diagnosis of schizoaffective disorder, alcohol abuse, and liver disease. He was residing in an apartment with limited case management support as he was always on a Medicaid spend down and could not access nursing services. He was living in an unsafe and unsanitary apartment where people were taking over the apartment and using alcohol. After going to a medical appointment, he was given nine months to live if he didn't get into treatment for alcohol abuse.

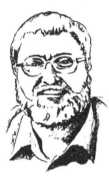

CURT

Curt is a forty-five-year-old Caucasian single male with a diagnosis of traumatic brain injury and a history of alcohol abuse. He received treatment and was discharged to the community with twenty-four-hour staffing in an independent apartment. He has a residential assistant, clinician, psychiatrist, behaviorist, substance abuse counselor, Department of Social Services case manager, Department of Mental Health worker, a representative from the Acquired Brain Injury Medicaid Waiver, a nursing home health aide, and conservator. He struggles with depression and isolation, and he sleeps most of the day when he has unstructured time.

CHAPTER 8 WORKSHOP FOR IMPLEMENTING AN INTERRELATED SERVICE SYSTEM

What follows is a short workshop designed over fifteen years as a tool to get you thinking about your agency, the degree to which you relate to others around you, and your system of care.

The workshop provides a framework for considering how you, one person, can help to change your own institutional culture, thus improving the way members of your work group, team, or agency interact. Change has to start from within. The questions are straightforward, but I suggest you not take them lightly. To complete the workshop sufficiently takes weeks and months, not minutes or even hours.

How many of the 7 Cs can you honestly say you have mastered? How willing are you to expose your work to the free and open commentary of your peers and your administration? If you're an administrator, how willing are you to acknowledge the shortcomings of your business model and reevaluate the principles of care that you've subscribed to for what could be decades?

You need to break some eggs to make egg salad. Go for it. Make a mess and rebuild in a spirit of collaboration. Take your time and envision the fruits of your work influencing not just you and your team but countless others. Design your system knowing that someday it will be bigger and better than anything you could have dreamed it would be.

I've done a lot of the legwork for you so don't reinvent the wheel. Also, don't try to go it alone. Pay close attention to important questions in the workshop and bring players on board who will work with you through the creation of a new and better system of care. This system is proactive and efficient in the spirit of collaboration.

STEP 1: EVALUATION

Is the culture of the organization such that members are willing to engage in introspection and to critically self-evaluate the need to improve qualitatively and continuously?

This is the foundational question in this step, but it will likely be the hardest question of all to answer. You can expect to wrestle with this one for a while.

For additional clarity, ask the following questions:

- *Do we have open-mindedness regarding new ideas?*

- *Are we willing to take risks?*

- *Does this willingness to grow and change extend to participation of all staff at all levels?*

- *Do we have systems in place to evaluate the risks we are taking and report on their efficacy?*

- *Who should we get input from regarding new opportunities and risks?*

- *Who is the ultimate decision maker regarding new ideas and practices here?*

- *What is that person's role in determining the organizational acceptance and adherence to policy and procedure?*

- *Have we given that person autonomy to thoroughly assess our programming and effectiveness?*

- *Are materials and opportunity for training and reviewing changes available?*

- *Will we want to collect data re new policies and procedures? How will this be done?*

STEP 2: COMMITMENT AND RESPONSIBILITIES

To what extent is the necessary administrative support available to achieve an Interrelated Service System? Is there administrative commitment within the program to create this type of system? If yes, ask these questions:

- *How is this commitment demonstrated?*
- *What else should be done?*
- *Is there "outside" commitment?*
- *Which agencies are likely to commit?*
- *Who has responsibility for ensuring that systems are interrelated and the fundamentals of these systems are applied uniformly within your program?*
- *Is there a liaison established to outside agencies?*
- *Where and when should meetings take place?*
- *Who is responsible for arranging meetings and setting agendas?*
- *Who should be included when contemplating steps necessary for ensuring consistent integration of services? (Start with the client and explore his or her wishes.)*

STEP 3: SERVICES NEEDED

To what extent does the program have a mechanism in place to determine what other agencies may be needed in order to facilitate a more interrelated approach for each client? Also ask these questions:

- *What services may be needed that are not or cannot be provided by your program?*
- *What agencies may be able to provide these services?*
- *How can you facilitate the services of these agencies in the areas of need?*

- *Who **must** be included in all aspects of services when planning for the benefit of a client?*

STEP 4: TRAINING ON OTHER AGENCIES AND SERVICES

To what extent should training be sought by program staff and administrators regarding other agencies and systems administration? Ask these questions:

- *Is program staff aware of the benefits outside agencies may bring?*
- *Is program staff aware of where they fit into the various life continuums of their clients?*
- *Is program staff aware of where other agencies fit into the various life continuums of their clients?*

STEP 5: POLICIES AND PROCEDURES

To what extent does the program have in place policies and procedures designed to facilitate an Interrelated Service System? Ask these questions:

- *Do policies address inclusion of outside agencies?*
- *Have policies been drafted to foster collaboration while considering issues of confidentiality?*
- *Do policies consider the wishes of the client and empower him/her to decide who is a participant?*
  - To what extent is this realistic?
  - What are the limitations of doing so (fiduciary, parole/probation vs. family and friends)?

- *Is a policy designed to collaboratively address possible crises?*
  - Who is included?
  - Who ought to be?
  - Who does the client want included?
- *To what extent are policies designed to be **collaborative**, foster **communication**, and ensure services are **coordinated** and **comprehensive**, and that **consistency** exists throughout the program?*

As you begin the journey of creating an Interrelated Service System, you're truly breaking old molds. You'll become a crusader and a *tour de force*. Make no mistake; this is a movement that will exponentially affect many thousands of lives.

The beauty of what you do is that you don't need to sell it. The concepts in this book aren't for sale like widgets or other products you might be convinced to buy. They spell out ways our systems need to change. The more people you reach with this Interrelated Service System, the more widely and readily change will be accepted. This approach to providing services to those in need is based on common sense and constitutes good practice.

CONCLUSION: MELISSA'S LEGACY

After a lot of tears and heartache, Melissa is thriving in the community. State mental health officials placed her in a specialized program. There, she could learn life skills and discover more about her illness and what would work best to control it. Naturally, she's not "cured" of mental illness, but she's learned coping mechanisms to assist her in times of need. To her credit, she has maintained an apartment for several years, stays out of the hospital, and last I heard, is engaged to be married.

Melissa's relationship with family members is good and they remain strong advocates. Her mom Robin stays in touch with me. She recently showed up at a fund-raising event we sponsored, and truth be told, I didn't recognize her when she grabbed me to give me a hug. Robin looks like a different person altogether. She has life in her eyes again and she carries herself comfortably. Long gone are the steely gazes and the puffed-up bravado of a woman at war with an entire system grappling with her daughter's mental illness.

This story is as much about Robin as it is about Melissa. And it's also about Melissa's sister, her boyfriend, her team of providers, her friends, and all her relatives. The tentacles of growth stretch infinitely beyond one person. So by supporting one individual, we help a host of others in turn.

Melissa touched me in a profound manner, allowing me to reach thousands of people directly and indirectly. I'm proud and grateful for this opportunity, for I've taken her story and turned it into my life's work. Because of her, a small nonprofit has received national recognition and accolades. We've won awards and speak about her legacy across the country.

Now you, too, can carry her torch.

APPENDIX A: SYSTEMS ISSUES

I would be remiss if I didn't mention several gripes I have with the mental health delivery system. Here's my chance to get on my soapbox. I welcome your reactions and comments.

LEAST RESTRICTIVE MEANS OF INTERVENTION

This phrase is all the rage in the law and ethics of caring for individuals who otherwise can't care for themselves. It seems straightforward enough; the amount of care we should provide is what's least invasive, much like determining elective surgery. But the issue becomes exponentially more complex as we discuss individuals who are mentally incapacitated and cannot or do not make informed decisions on their own.

Necessarily, the discussion needs to start there. What is the least restrictive means of intervention for an individual who is incapacitated in this way? Do we appoint a surrogate, a guardian, or a conservator? Do we trust the judgment of the individual to designate someone on his or her own? What should the role of the appointee be? What if we disagree with that person's decisions?

Indeed, is the appointment of a third-person decision maker the least restrictive means of intervention? Can an individual receive treatment or services without this intervention? Does a third party offer anything more to the overall treatment issues than would otherwise be provided in her or his absence?

This complex set of questions is at the core of intervening on behalf of individuals who are mentally incapacitated. Some contend that each person has the right to be mentally ill and we all have a right to make bad decisions. Of course, this leads back to the argument of "Least Restrictive Means of Intervention."

I readily concede that a fiduciary should only be assigned when that individual can bring value to the table. A fiduciary should not be present just for the sake of having another "warm body" or to offer comfort to a team member who doesn't want to make difficult decisions as dictated by his or her role or profession.

Bioethicist Viki Kind wrote an amazing book about the art of decision making for others. In *The Caregiver's Path to Compassionate Decision Making*, she masterfully breaks down the elements that must go into surrogate decision making. What an art! She dissects something we all do every day and exposes the processes involved in a manner that gives us pause to reconsider the reflex of that very action.

One standard Ms. Kind alludes to has already been identified and is the one most often applied in the field of mental health. The "Best Interest" standard is used when we don't know what a patient would want. Admittedly, it's the worst of the options of surrogate decision making. However, it's most often used in the realm of mental illness when we can't necessarily rely on the opinions of the individual we represent.

As a best practice in the world of mental health, we attempt to use a "Best Interest" standard coupled with a "Substituted Judgment" standard. Under the latter, we take what we know about the client and his or her preferences, and we make decisions based on that. We care what that individual wants (Substituted Judgment), and we strive to achieve that for him or her in a manner that's safe and reasonable (Best Interest). Such judgment requires a delicate balancing act of need versus desire, safety versus autonomy. (See Appendix C for a synopsis of the concepts of Guardianship/Conservatorship, which can be used as a reference guide for practitioners.)

The law helps us in this regard by offering the Least Restrictive standard, which suggests we tip the scales in favor of the wishes of the patient. However, least restrictive does not mean *not* restrictive, a mistake commonly made by advocates and frequently interpreted erroneously by courts. We all live with restrictions of one type or another.

The following case is an example.

K was in court complaining to the judge that she wasn't being allowed to move into the apartment of her choosing in a questionable part of town.

Care providers stated their concern that K, who had a history of prostitution and drug abuse, would be easily victimized in the community, would be unable to obtain food, and wouldn't use public transportation to meet with her clinicians and obtain the medications that would allow her to maintain independence.

The judge reasoned that K could have groceries delivered and that state agencies could create a program wherein she was provided with transportation to and from her apartment to see her clinician. Likewise, he reasoned that the agency could wrap her up with services to include nursing, medication monitoring, skill building, case management, and therapy groups, which would protect her from victimization. Therefore, the judge felt that to prevent her from moving into the apartment she wanted was to deny her the least restrictive level of care, and he approved of her request to move.

I was not afforded the opportunity to make a presentation that day due to my status as an observer in this matter. However, my argument to the judge, which may or may not have been persuasive, would have gone as follows:

> *"Your honor, K has a history of shutting out service providers. The programs you've described sound wonderful, but they don't exist right now. The state agency doesn't have the resources you identify, and even if it did, it's quite probable that K wouldn't avail herself of them. The alternative placement to that sought by K is least restrictive in that it's the only option currently available to meet her wishes AND keep her safe in the community."*

In other words, the judge's plan was neither **realistic** nor **attainable**.

It must be noted that "least restrictive" applies to both the physical residence of an individual as well as the treatment modalities used to address clinical needs.

Naturally, if given unlimited resources, we can create a system in which all the services perfectly match the needs of all our clients. There seems to be an inherent assumption that "least restrictive environment" means either one's home or independent living. The burden has been placed on decision makers and interested individuals to demonstrate that independent living is *not* the least restrictive.

However, that's not the reality of the Human Services field. Least restrictive does not absolutely mean completely independent living when the circumstances of a case warrant consideration of alternatives. The analysis needs to be approached from both sides, giving equal weight to protection, need, and best interest as well as the wishes of each individual, particularly where mental incapacity is a factor.

In my example, the court cautiously reviewed the case. It considered what the conserved person is capable of with *extraordinary* supports rather than what that individual is capable of under "normal" supports—standards of practice generally accepted in the mental health community.

There's a significant divergence here from the true intent of the law and the concept of least restrictive environment/means of intervention. In theory, the law protects individuals from being placed in an environment or a treatment modality that's more restrictive than that which they can reasonably manage without care from outside agencies. However, in practice, the law is being applied in a way that places undue burdens on social service agencies in our communities. *Not the least of these burdens is the "legal" burden of proving a client's capabilities to manage.*

When an agency thinks an individual cannot handle certain activities that would allow him or her to maintain independence, the current practice would be to request proof. In proving such, an agency would need to demonstrate to the court that the client had been receiving the required service from the agency, and when it was discontinued, the client was unable to acquire the same services independently. *However,* those services may not be available except with funding provided under state and local contracts. *Plus,* to remove a necessary service from a client simply to prove the client needs it and can't obtain it would be perilous to any agency, not to mention the person himself or herself.

The effect of this slippery slope is backing service agencies into a corner, which will be counterproductive to clinical treatment. Agencies are forced to allow clients to *fail* in order to secure from the courts what the agency has deemed to be clinically in the clients' best interest.

Also, agencies can't be expected to maintain extraordinary levels of care for individuals. In situations where service agencies are already acting well above the standard using internally established protocols, to assume they should continue to maintain that level of care at a cost to other consumers is flawed. Most often, agencies provide extra care for the short term, awaiting a long-term solution. To expect these agencies to continue to exceed what's commonly expected of them is to effectively punish them for doing so in the first place, and that's *not* what "least restrictive" means. In other words, the courts do not have the jurisdiction or the power to mandate that agencies provide extraordinary services to individuals in response to the argument that such services would allow individuals to remain in a least restrictive environment.

The creation of *new* protocols and the expectation that all services conceivable should be created to maintain a client in the community is a burden no service agency should be expected to carry.

Agencies can't be expected to *create* new protocols for treatment of *all* individuals for the sake of providing the least restrictive environment for *all* individuals. To mandate such would be to assume that every individual is *capable* of living in the least restrictive environment available to them (i.e., his/her own home). That is, as long as they're wrapped in services no service agency could hope to provide under the current culture or available funds and resources of the industry.

This translation will ultimately have the effect of freezing all services currently being afforded to individuals in need. It's entirely foreseeable that no new programming will be created due to the burden of meeting the standards already in place.

Furthermore, under the translations being adopted by the courts, a client in clinical need of a more restrictive course of treatment (including residence) isn't likely to receive it in the future.

Cutting through all of the legalese, I'm arguing that third-party decisions can't be made in a vacuum.

Unfortunately, we have to deal with the reality of the individual *and* the limitations of systems of care to define least restrictive means of intervention and least restrictive environment. We don't live in a fantasy world with unrestricted resources. Otherwise, we'd have no need to stress the standard of Least Restriction, as it would always be defined as the sum total of everything available to all patients at all times under all circumstances.

I wish I could live in that world.

ENGAGEMENT

It's a well-established tenet of social work and human services practice and, indeed, a basic principle in all human interaction: *Rapport needs to be established to build and maintain any meaningful relationship.* Barriers to rapport are many and varied. Likewise, rapport can be established using many different techniques and best practices (Hepworth, 1997). However it's achieved, engagement on a level that's comfortable to the individual is of paramount importance to the work of the social services fields.

In their comprehensive work "Disengagement from Mental Health Services," Aileen O'Brien et al determined the following as possible barriers to engagement:

- *Gender – Women tend to engage more than men (O'Brien et al 2008)*.[5]

- *Age – Young people seem to be more difficult to engage and more likely to drop services than older people.*

- *Ethnicity – Minorities tend to engage less than Caucasians with mental health services.*

- *Dual diagnosis – Individuals who are diagnosed with a mental illness and some form of substance abuse.*

- *Insight into illness – To what extent does the individual acknowledge he/she has an illness, is motivated to address it, and empowered to make changes.*

- *Stage of illness – ". . . the most frequent outpatient appointment not attended is the first one"* [6]

- *Attitude/experience of caregivers – The extent to which the provider is invested and shows empathy and knowledge of systems/services combined with an individual's needs.*

- *Unemployment*

- *Lack of education*

- *Low income*

- *Low social class*

- *Lack of health insurance*

- *Social deprivation – Determination if the individual has friends, family and a network of social supports.*

- *Living alone, separated, divorced, without family*

- *Homelessness*

- *Lack of communication skills or tools*

- *Forensic history – Determination if the individual been involved in criminal activity as a result of or related to his/her illness and manifestations that follow.*

- *Borderline Personality Disorder – over-represented (40%). (Schizophrenia is the opposite, especially if engaged within six months.)*

The term "rapport" or more commonly "engagement" has many definitions and can be quite subjective when viewed on a case-by-case basis. Indeed, a simple nod or smile may be a huge leap for one client, while a friendly lunch or cup of coffee may be engagement in the mind of another. To be sure, engagement goes far beyond medication compliance, telephone conversations, or caseworkers allowed into one's home.

Engagement encompasses all the terms and concepts commonly recognized in the therapeutic setting and more. We can consider engagement based on the willingness of a client to work on clearly identified goals along with a caseworker, counselor, or other professional.

Interestingly, the strong therapeutic relationship described herein is not only helpful in generating engagement, but is also a by-product thereof (M. Gillespie et al 2004). Here we see that engagement is not only a process but must also be seen as a service provided (O'Brien et al 2008). Still, it's common for one to be "engaged" as part of a process but maintain ill feelings toward the therapist or professional or the entire service system. Thus, a better working definition of engagement may be taken from O'Brien et al:

> *[Engagement] is a more complex phenomenon encompassing factors that include acceptance of a need for help, the formation of a therapeutic alliance with professionals, satisfaction with the help already received and a mutual acceptance and working toward shared goals. (O'Brien et al 2008, 559)*

In defining engagement, O'Brien et al recognize that "physical presence or attendance is necessary" to the process but is clearly not the only element to the service associated with engagement (O'Brien et al 2008, 559).

O'Brien et al recognize the need for metrics to discern the appropriate level of engagement among and within certain demographics (2008). Some may have more socioeconomic reasons for not engaging or disengaging, while others may be experiencing clinical factors or socio-demographic factors that preclude engagement. Significantly, many may be experiencing the manifestations of their particular illnesses when they "choose" not to engage. In any event, "engagement is one of several *essential* components identified in case management approaches." (A. Paget et al 2009, 74)

Indeed, lack of engagement has been cited as an indicator of the likelihood of involvement with more intensive services to include criminal involvement and hospitalization. Early engagement has been found to indicate a likelihood of continued participation in therapy, medication compliance, and longer periods of stability (Gillespie et al, 2004). Further, engagement has been shown to increase over time and can remain stable for many years. This is clearly an important factor when, as discussed, the relationship and "service" of engagement acts as a foundation for many other therapeutic approaches and interventions. (A. Paget et al 2009)

AWARENESS OF MENTAL ILLNESS

Awareness is addressed here in two ways. First, awareness is something promoted globally by people who have romantic notions of the ability to inform society of its ills. Awareness in this regard is a call to action, a movement of almost spiritual proportions. "Say NO to Drugs," "Click it or Ticket," or "No means No." Let's call this Macro Level awareness—awareness on a big level.

Second, awareness is knowledge about something. It's that simple. Did you know there's a system of care that can provide medical coverage for you if you're unable to afford it? Did you know that a red-tailed hawk is more closely related to an owl than a true hawk? Did you know a giraffe is the tallest animal on the planet? Let's call this type of awareness Micro Level because it relates to an individual's knowledge.

MACRO LEVEL AWARENESS

It makes me crazy when I hear advocates waxing poetic about reducing stigma around mental illness. No stigma was ever reduced
by simply saying we were going to reduce it. Slavery has been abol-
ished, women have the vote, gay people serve in the military, and
the Special Olympics raises millions of dollars for kids with developmental disabilities.

Reducing stigma requires societal change such as these examples. And creating societal change takes work.

Social work as an entity came about, not surprisingly, in the
1960s. Its original design looked nothing like it does today—and
this isn't good. Economic forces and politics have resulted in a
system that's been beaten down almost irreparably. An institution once designed to address the needs of the individual now
applauds itself when it comes up with new terms to express old
ideas, such as "person-centered planning," "harm reduction,"
"trauma informed," "recovery oriented," and "the ecological approach." This is sad because true social work can't be designed in
cookie-cutter fashion and spouted like ingredients in a cookbook.
By its nature, *social work needs to be iterative and individualized.*

Stigma can be reduced over years of hard work by dedicated
people who care deeply. Society has beaten down social work to
a shadow of what it once was, but it's the last great hope to dispel
stigma in our communities. Removing stigma is a social change;
it's not a slogan or an empty affirmation.

To create social change starts with an audience. In countless
presentations to thousands across the country, I have continued to
ask not only for money but also for a wider audience. This message needs to get out: *The issues that face those living with and working
with mental illnesses are still "in the closet" of our social conscience.* Awareness is increasing, but we have a long way to go.

MICRO LEVEL AWARENESS

Most of the people I speak to already know problems out there need to be addressed. They don't realize that a lot of people with those problems don't know they have problems that need to be addressed. Even if they do know they have problems, they don't know where to turn to address them.

Perhaps the first hurdle to overcome, as care providers, family members, coordinators, and/or clients of human service systems, is knowing a "system" even exists. This ignorance isn't limited to a certain socioeconomic standing, ethnicity, culture, and more. People who are rich and poor, smart and stupid, may have a family member affected by mental illness. It's estimated mental illness impacts between five to ten percent of people in the United States. These numbers don't take into consideration those who are embarrassed by their illness, have mild forms of it, or simply don't know they have issues.

Mental illness doesn't discriminate. It doesn't care if you're black or white, gay or straight, wealthy or destitute. Some of the most sophisticated, educated, and well-off people have no idea there's an entire community of people there to help them and their loved ones navigate the systems of care. Not stupid or closed-minded, they simply had never had a reason to think about mental illness.

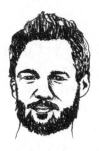

MATTHEW'S STORY

Consider the case of Matthew, the son of a wealthy land developer. Matt and his family had never experienced mental health issues. All members of this wealthy family had attended prestigious colleges and universities. They had no reason to know of the services available to them as a family and individually for treatment of psychiatric and substance use disorders.

One day, Matthew decided his father was a satanic cult leader who needed to be "taught a lesson." He locked the garage of their palatial home, and after luring his father inside, proceeded to beat him for almost an hour.

Luckily, Matt's father survived after suffering a subdural hematoma and undergoing hours of brain surgery. It wasn't until this event that the family was forced to get help for their adult son. Then came the monumental task of finding that help.

Matt was lucky enough to have parents who cared for him and could research areas of the mental health system. Still, despite their considerable wealth and sophistication, Matt's family found the system to be overwhelming, confusing, and disjointed. Being immersed in a system that is, by definition, exclusionary, people feel overwhelmed trying to fit into the "big picture."

Often, family members aren't welcome participants at all. Providers tend to overlook the valuable historical data a family can offer. Also, family members may be seen as intrusive or even an obstacle to recovery. Providers might even feel tentative due to HIPAA regulations.

RECOVERY

For a long time, there was a movement sweeping the country that defined the way systems of care should relate to their clients. The Recovery movement was 1) a proponent of all things least restrictive, 2) honored client choice above all other considerations, and 3) recognized the ability of all individuals to self-determine what a "meaningful life" is to them.

Here is how I respond to the Recovery movement:

1. *As far as "least restrictive" is concerned, see comments on pages 101–106.*

2. *Clients have the right to make bad choices, but a fiduciary has a mandated responsibility to make smart, best-interest choices where a court of law has determined the individual is incapable of doing so.*

3. *Some clients are so beset with mental illness, they can't make informed decisions about what a meaningful life is for them.*

Consider the case of J:

J wanted to be released from the hospital and he told his doctor this as well as his lawyer. His lawyer advocated that if J says he wants out, the doctor and the hospital must release him.

The doctor and hospital and I argued that J was not making this decision with a clear understanding of what it truly meant because he was impaired by his mental illness. He would be released from the hospital with no clothing except what he was wearing, no shelter, and no community-based services. In all likelihood, J would be back in an emergency room within a day or two—or he would die.

If he had the capacity to understand this, J would certainly not push for release from the hospital.

Here we used the combination of Substituted Judgment and Best Interest standard of decision making for J. I submit that, above all else, we were really using a Reasonable Person standard here, masterfully described by Viki Kind (see References), but is considered a part of the Best Interest standard rather than a standard unto itself.

In fact, instead of subscribing to the concept of a recovery-oriented system of care, I believe we should subscribe to this combination of Best Interest/Reasonable Person standard. This is particularly true where Substituted Judgment is ruled out due to the severity of the individual's mental incapacity.

THE STUPIDITY DEFENSE

The stupidity defense is used when providers, for a number of reasons, go out of their way to allow individuals who are acutely psychotic to make choices that are clearly not in their own best interests or may even be dangerous to themselves or others. This position contends that those beset with chronic illnesses have the right to make wrong choices, even when they can't help themselves because they're so ill. It does not consider that people also have the right to be healthy and make choices that a healthy mind would make.

In fact, this isn't a matter of their *right* to make a bad decision. It's a matter of their *ability* to make a decision at all when every decision is compromised due to an illness. This creates an ethical argument in which the only answer on one side is to allow individuals to "die with their rights on." In other words, "Why should we care if a person is making horrible decisions on their own behalf as long as we recognize their right to do so?"

It just doesn't make sense in a discussion of the ethical treatment of those who've been deemed incapable of caring for themselves. It's an unfortunate reality, but there are people out there who need the help of all of us as a society. To cast aside that help and offer the excuse that privacy laws prevail, or civil liberties prevail, or individual dignity prevails is to ignore the issue altogether.

Probate courts in this country have long been given jurisdiction over mental incapacity. For hundreds of years, we've stood by the tenet that government has a duty to oversee the care of those who cannot care for themselves. This includes children who are deemed to lack the mental capacity for responsible decision making and the elderly patient suffering from dementia. It should extend to persons with mental illnesses.

Historically, the process has been painful and is wrought with horrifying stories of abuse and neglect on the part of court-appointed fiduciaries. However, we have an historical basis to justify the appointment of surrogate decision makers. This can and should be embraced as a clinical tool to assist the team of providers in collaboratively arriving at a decision made in the best interest of the mutual client or patient.

APPENDIX B: GENERAL PROBATE COURT PROCESS

An interrelated system of care depends heavily on an involved probate court, which has jurisdiction over the majority of the populations most at need in our communities. We've found that judges are receptive to the idea of monitoring those with mental illness more closely and acting as an ever-watchful eye over them. Clients naturally respond to the wishes of the probate court judge, as he or she is seen not only as an authority figure who genuinely cares for their well-being but also as an important individual interested in the issues they face daily. This mutual respect creates an atmosphere of cooperation, and positive results typically follow.

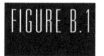 **FIGURE B.1** The Revolving Door Between Treatment and Community

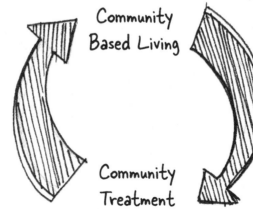

Community Based Living

Community Treatment

COMMUNITY-BASED LIVING

We've identified cyclical patterns in the lives of those with mental illness and have labeled it "the revolving door." In its most basic form, the revolving door involves a client who's in need of community-based mental health services but manages to live in the community with any number of providers involved peripherally or intensively in their lives. Treatment of mental illness is a balance between this community-based living and community-based treatment. Ideally, the individual is the center of the planning for treatment, setting his/her own goals of recovery and identifying wishes for fulfillment. In our experience, the best model of community-based treatment is person-centered case management, as opposed to the stricter medical model that some agencies adhere to.

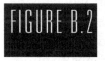 The Revolving Door
Involving Decompensation

Community
Based Living

Decompensation

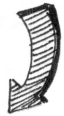

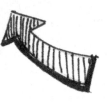

Community
Treatment

DECOMPENSATION

Decompensation is sometimes expected in the lives of the chronically mentally ill. Unfortunately, persons with mental illnesses may experience lapses in the delivery of needed services or, as is often the case, may not receive the appropriately prescribed medication for their treatment and begin a slow or rapid period of decompensation. At times, individuals refuse to take their medications for a variety of reasons, including real and perceived side effects or simple negligence. Decompensation can be gradual or, in some instances, quite rapid. It's the job of the case manager, physician, and Crisis Intervention to *react* to decompensation as there hasn't traditionally been a mechanism in place to treat decompensation proactively.

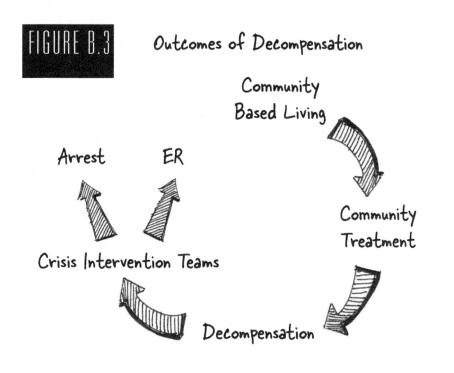

FIGURE B.3 Outcomes of Decompensation

Community Based Living

Community Treatment

Decompensation

Crisis Intervention Teams

Arrest

ER

CRISIS INTERVENTION

Decompensation leads us to three potential outcomes. First, the crisis can be de-escalated, the individual can be redirected, and the proscribed treatment plan can be continued with minor adjustments if necessary. Second, decompensation can lead to criminal behaviors that leave authorities no choice but to detain an individual for his/her own safety and the safety of others. Finally, decompensation can lead to hospitalization, involuntary commitment, and the process we describe as the Probate Court Revolving Door.

Decompensation and subsequent hospitalization should not always be perceived as a "bad thing." Hospitalization often gives an individual a much-needed respite from the stressors of his/her symptomology and is often the endgame in their struggle against the overwhelming manifestations of illness. Likewise, it affords the organized, cohesive treatment team the opportunity to "regroup," candidly discuss the shortcomings of the treatment plan, and collaboratively implement corrective actions on the part of responsible parties.

Ideally, hospitals will be included in crisis planning, and Crisis Alert Protocols (CAP) will be developed for those who are high users of the services in community-based medical centers. CAP is a program that's part of The Guardian Model. It sets off a chain or web of communication to advise all treatment personnel of the current crisis facing individuals, and is often the launching point for the collaboration described above. Further, it's important to include local authorities in CAP planning so individuals exhibiting the manifestations of mental illness are directed to an appropriate medical center or ER for treatment. It's vitally important to differentiate between the manifestation of illness and criminality and/or criminal intent at the outset of planning and response during crisis.

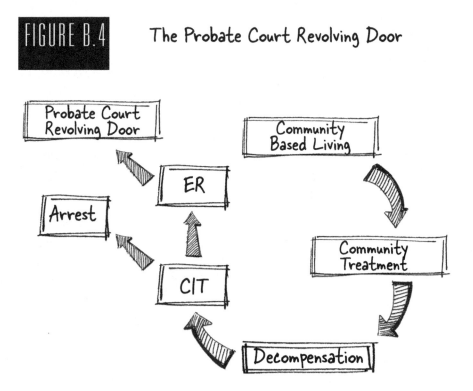

FIGURE B.4 The Probate Court Revolving Door

EMERGENCY HOSPITALIZATION

When it's determined an individual needs prolonged hospitalization due to the severity of his/her illness or the depth to which he/she has decompensated, the hospital must file the appropriate application for involuntary commitment. (This assumes that a physician's emergency certificate is expiring.)

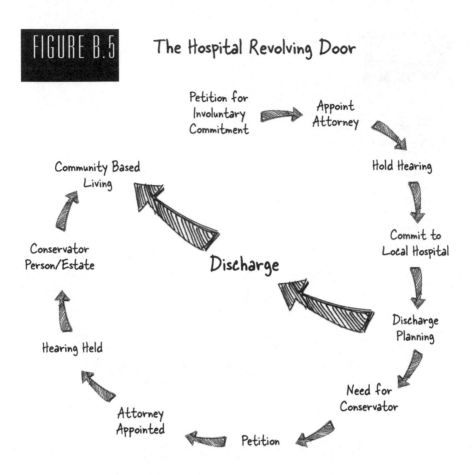

FIGURE B.5   The Hospital Revolving Door

INVOLUNTARY COMMITMENT

Upon receipt of this application, the probate court must schedule a hearing and appoint an attorney for the individual who's the subject of the petition. This attorney is referred to as the "attorney for respondent" (AFR). It's the AFR's responsibility to gather facts regarding issues leading up to the hospitalization, the structure and services available to his/her client in the community, and the desires of the client relative to the application, among other pertinent factors.

A formal hearing is held, usually at the facility proposed as the place for involuntary commitment. At that time, the respondent must be afforded all due process rights, including the right to cross-examine any witnesses. The burden is on the petitioner or applicant, usually the hospital, to prove by clear and convincing evidence that the respondent should be involuntarily committed to the facility because he/she is gravely disabled and/or a danger to self or others, or no less restrictive placement is available in the community.

It's vitally important that the petitioner and his/her witnesses have intimate details of the issues facing the respondent. In other words, the petitioner(s) must show that, despite their best efforts and the use of a multitude of resources and corrective planning, the respondent needs to be confined against his/her will.

Having made the appropriate findings in a recorded, formal evidentiary hearing, the judge of probate has the ability to involuntarily commit the individual to the facility. Under The Guardian Model, discharge planning would begin immediately upon receipt of this notice. Such planning would once again involve all of the individuals potentially involved in the life of the respondent/patient and would seek to implement realistic attainable plans for sustaining meaningful life in the community.

It's interesting. Strong language dictates under what circumstances an individual may be involuntarily committed to a facility. However, little guidance and no prescribed oversight are available as to the discharge of an individual back into the community.

When a patient is prematurely discharged or detained for a period longer than is warranted, the patient is harmed by the very people allegedly assisting him or her. The patient must be the center for all of this, which should start with communication and planning around his/her basis of reality, wishes, and goals.

Hopefully, treatment in the facility will have met with success, and discharge planning will be implemented in the form of a community-based treatment plan. The individual will return to meaningful life in the community—whatever that may mean to each one.

Unfortunately, all too often discharge/treatment plans aren't cohesive and aren't arrived at collaboratively. Thus individuals are discharged under the same plan that resulted in their hospital-ization in the first place, and the process of decompensation may begin all over again.

APPENDIX C: BASIC CONSERVATORSHIP GUIDE

APPLICATION FOR CONSERVATORSHIP

Very often in the revolving door process described in Appendix B, it's determined that no third party is available to assist the team in reaching consensus for a plan. Given the appropriate characteristics of each case, the hospital or other interested party may deem it appropriate to file an application for Involuntary Appointment of a Conservator. (*Note:* an individual need not be hospitalized for an interested party to make an application for such appointment.) The laws that apply to this appointment and the responsibilities of individuals assigned to this fiduciary responsibility have drastically changed throughout the years. An exploration of the important facets of conservatorship, as well as an evaluation of the changes in law, follow.

As in the Involuntary Commitment Process, an attorney is appointed to represent the individual to be conserved (the "respondent") and is, again, referred to as Attorney for Respondent. The attorney representing an individual in a commitment hearing is not necessarily the individual appointed to represent him/her in a conservator proceeding.

A formal hearing on the application will be held after legal notice to interested parties. At this hearing, a physician's evaluation is required, which details the current condition of the respondent including the reasons he or she needs a conservator, if appropriate. Interestingly, the current statutes indicate specifically that the respondent has the right to refuse a physician's evaluation. In this case, the court must be made aware of the refusal and make a finding that the evaluation has been waived. Presumably, such refusal should not be taken as *prima facie* evidence of the need for a conservator. The court is then left to rely on testimony from caseworkers, family and other relations, Department of Social Services, case management, coordinating, assessment and monitoring agencies, etc. It then must consider other relevant reports and factors.

Similarly, if he indicates a preference, the respondent should be allowed to choose an attorney he wishes to represent him in the matter. If he can't afford an attorney, a court-appointed attorney will be paid from funds established by the Office of the Probate Court Administrator. Whenever possible, courts accommodate the wishes of the respondent in appointing an attorney of choice. Of course, the respondent may refuse to be represented by an attorney.

CONSERVATORSHIP

Generally speaking, it's the job of a conservator to "conserve." We expect, in fact mandate to a degree, that a conservator conserve the assets, property, real and otherwise, and even the "person" of their "ward" to the extent possible. The conservator is ultimately acting as an agent of the court and is therefore accountable to it. There are forms for reporting on the condition of the conserved person by a court-appointed conservator of the person as well as regular requirements thereto. Further, the conservator of estate is required to account for his/her doings relative to assets of the conserved person once every three years at minimum.

Conservators are entitled to reimbursement for their time spent to the extent that they submit the requisite forms to the Probate Court Administration *and* they are among the group of parties entitled to reimbursement. For instance, family members of an indigent person are not typically reimbursed for their efforts as conservator. In the event that a conserved person has assets and the ability to pay, family members and independent third-party conservators are allowed reimbursement at a rate commensurate with their respective "position" and experience in such matters. The rate of compensation in these matters varies from court to court and should be approved therein prior to payment.

The appointment of a conservator, in my opinion and experience, is the greatest taking of personal liberties available under our civil laws. It's not a fiduciary position or responsibility that should be taken lightly or entered into without careful consideration of one's ability to undertake the challenges. Money is hardly an appropriate consideration for accepting or denying the fiduciary appointment.

A conserved person should retain all decision-making rights that are not expressly removed or assigned to a conservator. Historically, we considered that the conservator figuratively "stepped into the shoes of the conserved person," or the conservator "became the conserved person for all intents and purposes." For instance, a conservator of person, by virtue of his/her appointment, assumed responsibility for all health-care decisions, the residence, and daily needs of his/her ward. Likewise, a conservator of estate was expected to assume control of all of the assets of the conserved person, even to the extent of filing a notice on the land records indicating that he was duly appointed, and any real property of the conserved person was not subject to sale without it first passing through the conservator (and the court). While this may still be required, one can presumably be appointed conservator of estate over certain assets and not others.

The courts today should, quite literally, develop checklists, not unlike the typical power of attorney form used in many circumstances, which clearly state what a conservator is or is not capable of doing on behalf of the conserved person. As always, contracts entered into by a conserved person are "voidable," not necessarily "void."

One of the most significant "findings" the court must make in determining the appropriateness of the designation of conservator is whether or not such designation is the least restrictive means of intervention. That is, "intervention for a conserved person that is sufficient to provide, within the resources available to the conserved person either from the conserved person's own estate or from private or public assistance, for a conserved person's personal needs, or property management while affording the conserved person the greatest amount of independence and self-determination."[7] This definition has already been the sticking point of many conservator hearings. Judges struggle with creative arguments in determining any number of factors, which, in a perfect world, would or should be available in the community for the care and maintenance of the respondent. Quite often, the expectations these judges place upon community providers to develop new programs around the needs of one client are not only inappropriate and beyond the judge's jurisdiction, but they are often unrealistic and untenable. Granted, given unlimited resources and finances, any of us can design the perfect program for care in the community for even the most difficult cases. However, quite often, the lack of funding and the lack of cooperation on the part of the respondent leave treatment providers with few realistic choices and paths of treatment.

The general focus has changed subtly but with great significance. We no longer focus on the factors that prevent an individual from maintaining activities of daily living. For instance, it's not enough to contend that an individual is in need of a conservator because she/he has a mental illness that prevents her/him from leaving the home and obtaining food and groceries.

Now, our inquiry must focus on that which an individual is *capable of* in determining the appropriateness of appointing an involuntary conservator and assigning the duties thereto. Again, our client may be quite capable, despite paranoia, of arranging for and allowing meal delivery to the home, thus accomplishing the task of providing for daily nutrition needs.

Although at first glance this language may seem to be a matter of semantics, the necessary inquiry and resultant findings based thereupon are quite significant. This is particularly true where, as described above, treatment providers have exhausted their resources, but a creative court develops an untenable opinion as to actions or treatments that should be attempted to allow the individual the ability to manage personal affairs. The result is a stalemate that's clinically inappropriate for the respondent.

JURISDICTION

The first obvious question pertaining to jurisdiction relates to the location of the respondent in all matters. Where is he/she now? Where is his/her domicile? (Where does he/she live?) Note that the only legal term in this inquiry is that of *domicile.*

Many of our courts are at odds internally with respect to continuing jurisdiction of conserved individuals who have been hospitalized in a facility outside of their jurisdiction—e.g., in hospital-based involuntary commitment issues as well as involuntary medication cases. Presently, there's no clear direction and these matters are addressed when proactive judges take it upon themselves to set a policy in this regard.

This open-endedness has led to much controversy. For instance, assume that an individual was conserved in BlackAcre and is now hospitalized in BlueAcre. Which judge has continuing jurisdiction over the conservator matter if issues are brought to the court? Which judge should hear involuntary commitment or involuntary medication controversies? These are seemingly straightforward under the new statutes, but the answers have, at times, been controversial between judges, petitioners, and family members.

Conspicuously omitted from statutes is a preference list as to the whereabouts of the respondent to guide the courts on matters regarding the proper court of jurisdiction.

Much of this line of questioning was exemplified in a Connecticut case that ultimately decided and sealed the fate of conservatorship when it went to Connecticut Supreme Court (Gross vs. Rell, 485 F.Supp.2d 72, 2007). In that matter, an elderly gentleman visiting from Long Island was conserved by a local court and was placed in a nursing home in Connecticut, resulting in the loss of interest or value in real and personal property. The controversial rulings, in this and many other cases centered on the protection of the elderly, were well-intended under these statutes. However, one can only begin to imagine their practical application outside of the courtroom and the congressional chambers creating them, particularly in the realm of mental health.

The Gross vs. Rell case contemplated the extension of judicial immunity for conservators in Connecticut, but the underlying facts of the case pose universal issues for consideration. Its key finding was that a conservator/guardian does not enjoy the same protection for the actions of a conserved person as does a judge. That is, the judge's judicial immunity does not extend to a fiduciary he/she has appointed for the care and maintenance of an individual. The only time this may not be true is if the fiduciary is carrying out specific orders made by the court.

The implications should be obvious. When a judge appoints a fiduciary, checks must be in place to ensure an individual is protected from abuse by that fiduciary. However, the fiduciary is not afforded protections under the law and may be held accountable for his/her actions and potentially the actions of the conserved individual.

In a system that's increasingly difficult to find willing and capable participants to act in a fiduciary role, this finding (and the slippery slope it creates) may result in making this process even more difficult. A thankless task becomes more difficult and risky for those who otherwise would be inclined to serve.

COURT FINDINGS

In considering the application for involuntary appointment of a conservator, the judge must consider factors to include those given and others. Again, in keeping with the themes of a recovery-oriented mental health-care system, much emphasis is placed upon client choice and preference when determining who should be a conservator. Likewise, much emphasis is placed upon the respondent's past practices, culture, and choice. Such consideration will also be given when determining *whom* the court will appoint.

Arguably, if an individual manages quite capably to obtain medical attention from means other than that which would be afforded by the appointment of a conservator, a fiduciary should not be appointed. This seems like an obvious statement, however, consider the individual with mental illnesses who presents to the emergency room fifteen times in one month claiming a sore arm, only to be sent home by the attending physician. Here, this gentleman was not medically compromised, but he was clearly experiencing instability as it related to his mental health. In this very real situation, a conservator may be clinically appropriate in an effort to assist the individual in making and adhering to a proper care plan or to arrange for proper assessment via collaboration with community providers.

In considering present supports available to the respondent, courts are emphasizing that state and private entities can, and probably should, be doing more, per contractual and statutory mandates.

Arguably, supportive services, technologies, or other means of assistance are *always* available somewhere, and the savvy attorney for the respondent can make, and has been making, this argument to receptive courts. Again, this is a slippery slope, and probate courts should not attempt to become involved. Theirs is not to dictate or order treatment planning. Nor should courts try to discern the limited resources of other state and private agencies or their uses thereof.

Of course, advance directives should be followed where and when appropriate to protect the best interest of individuals and to honor their dignity and respect their wishes.

In practical application, advance directives are not always useful in the case of persons with mental illnesses. The concept of creating advance directives, crisis plans, or a Wellness Recovery Action Plan (WRAP®, developed by the Copeland Center)is quite recovery-oriented and seeks to emphasize client choice. In its purest sense, the advance directive will be created by the individual in contemplation of his/her future incapacity and/or decompensation. Ideally, individuals will have prescribed the manner of treatment, the individuals to be involved, the hospital preferred, those to be notified, etc. However, at the moment when advance directives are most needed (i.e., during acute crisis) persons with mental illnesses often revoke them and indicate a wish not to be treated by anyone, not even those indicated in their original plans. In sticking with the concepts of recovery and honoring the rights and wishes of all individuals, we must adhere to their wishes even at the time of crisis. There is, as of yet, no recognized advance directive that will withstand the future incapacity of the maker other than the durable power of attorney and designation of conservator.

CLEAR AND CONVINCING EVIDENCE

Let's assume the court determines it has jurisdiction to hear the case and finds by clear and convincing evidence that the respondent is incapable of managing his/her affairs. The court must *also* consider whether these affairs can be managed without the appointment of a conservator and whether such an appointment is the least restrictive means of intervention.

Each matter will, of course, be considered and determined on a case-by-case basis.

DEFINING "INCAPABLE"

Incapable of caring for oneself was somewhat clearly defined in the past, although the practical application of the definition was difficult. To determine an "incapable" state, the question to ask was this: Does an individual have a mental, emotional, or physical condition that

- *results from mental illness, mental deficiency, physical illness or disability, chronic use of drugs or alcohol, or confinement, or*

- *results in the person's inability to provide medical care or physical and mental health needs, etc., or*

- *results in endangerment that causes him/her to be unable to meet essential requirements of personal needs because he/she cannot receive and evaluate information or communicate decisions, even if he/she has appropriate assistance?*

Significant is the addition of the language regarding appropriate assistance. This opens up a Pandora's box of possibilities and interpretations and wants for an exact definition of "appropriate assistance." Once again, we see an obvious abyss that courts may fall into as they independently try to define this amorphous phraseology.

CONSERVATOR DUTIES AND RESPONSIBILITIES

As indicated earlier, the general principle behind the designation of conservator is to conserve not only the assets but also the "person" of one's ward in the best manner possible. A conservator is clearly a benefit to the "state" and, as a matter of public policy, the designation of a conservator for individuals makes sense from a cost-savings perspective. Like Medicaid, it's clear that the work of a conservator can benefit and maintain an individual's independence and reliance on public assistance in the community for a longer period than would otherwise be possible. As a result, society saves dollars in the long run because the cost of institutional care is so high that it becomes prohibitive.

However, as mentioned before, conservatorship is not and should not be a dictatorship. While it means the usurping of civil liberties by a court of proper jurisdiction, it's limited to the purpose of protecting individuals. There's nothing punitive about conservatorship. The opinions, wants, needs, and goals of the conserved person should always be the paramount consideration when making decisions impacting him/her.

As an arm of the court, the conservator maintains a duty to report his/her activities relative to the conserved person as well as the person's condition, and to report the ongoing need (or not) of a conservator. Naturally, the conservator may have a duty to consent to medical treatment for the conserved person when appropriate. Along with this duty may come the duty of general custody of the conserved person: the duty to provide care, comfort, and maintenance to the person and care for his/her personal belongings—but otherwise undefined.

One of the trickiest aspects of conservatorship centers on the duty of establishing residence. This issue has always been one of concern for an appointed conservator, for it's clear no one can "force" an adult individual, conserved or otherwise, to live someplace he/she doesn't wish to live.

In requesting court permission to move an individual, the conservator must inform the court why the move is necessary. The conservator must also provide an explanation of the interventions attempted to avoid a new placement and the reasons the conserved person's needs can't be met in the community. Two notes: First, it's nearly impossible for a layperson, attorney, or others not in the field to comprehend the myriad resources available and entitlements of those who live in the community. Second, the system of housing is one of the most backlogged and undersupplied resources available to community providers. In the event a "bed" is secured for an individual, having to await the blessing of the proper probate court can be clinically catastrophic.

Finally, in attempting to prevent a move on behalf of a client as well as the probate court judge, it's presumed the court-appointed attorney for the respondent is fully aware of

- *all resources available,*
- *all resources that have been utilized or attempted,*
- *the degree to which a conserved person has availed or is willing to avail himself/herself of the services, and*
- *what is meant by a "Less Restrictive and More Integrated" environment.*

To be sure, none of these elements are easily defined.

Due to this lack of clarity, it becomes the burden of the conservator and treatment providers to advocate for a change in placement or oppose the request of the conserved person to be moved. This can clinically compromise the entire treatment continuum and calls for a shift in the burden when the conserved person is the petitioner.

TERMINATION OF CONSERVATORSHIP

Conservatorship ends upon the death of the conserved person. The conservator has no more authority to act in any manner and leaves all decisions to the decedent's executor or court-appointed administrator. A conservatorship can also be terminated by act of law, such as the restoration of the individual after a hearing. Again, the burden falls on the conserved person in a restoration hearing. But in practice, it shifts to any opposing party wishing to continue the conservatorship to present convincing evidence why the action to terminate should not be taken.

I am from Connecticut, which is on the forefront of mental health care in the United States. The fiduciary rules noted here are generalized to the extent they can/should be. The laws pertaining to conservatorship were drastically changed in 2007 to create relationships that are more recovery oriented, driven by least restrictive inquiries, and considerate of protecting and preserving the rights of a conserved individual. Still, many aspects of our laws have yet to be challenged; they simply do not work in a complex and overburdened mental health system.

However, the overarching message in these changes is sound. Conservatorship never was nor should it ever be a "dictatorship." Rather, it must be a collaborative relationship that's respectful of the dignity and basic human needs/rights of the conserved individual.

I also believe that conservatorship and its associated laws and policies can be used as a meaningful tool in the clinical treatment of persons with mental illnesses. It's unfortunate that, individually and as a society, we need to care for others. But we must approach that reality with our eyes open and apply our best intentions and understanding of how we're appointed to serve others.

REFERENCES

Arya, Dinesh, and Tom Callaly. "Using continuous quality improvement to implement a clinical governance framework in a mental health service." 13(3): *Australasian Psychiatry.* doi:10.1111/j.1440-1665.2005.02193.x, 2005.

Bolman, L. G., and T. E. Deal. *Reframing Organizations: Artistry, Choice, and Leadership.* San Francisco: Jossey-Bass, 2008.

Brassard, M., & D. Ritter. *The Memory Jogger II: A Pocket Guide of Tools for Continuous Improvement & Effective Planning.* New Hampshire: Goal/QPC. New Hampshire: Goal/QPC, 1994.

GM, and MJ Lambert. "Pragmatics of tracking mental health outcomes in a managed care setting." Academic Search Premier database: *Journal of Mental Health Administration, 22,3 (1995): 226-236.*

Carr-Leroy, K. *The 8-Step Continuous Improvement Model* [Power Point Presentation]. Retrieved from http://www.docfoc.com/the-8-step-continuous-improvement-model, 2016.

Cohen, Deborah J., et al. *A Guidebook for Professional Practices for Behavioral Health and Primary Care Integration: Observations from Exemplary Sites.* Rockville, MD: Agency for Healthcare Research and Quality, 2015.

Council of State Governments Justice Center Project (2002–
  2010). *The Consensus Project Report.* The CSG Justice Center.
  Retrieved from: https://csgjusticecenter.org/mental-health-
  projects/report-of-the-consensus-project/, 2002.

Department of Mental Health and Addiction Services
  (CT-DMHAS). *Consumer Survey-Satisfaction* (CS1).
  Hartford, Connecticut, May 2010.

Department of Mental Health and Addiction Services (CT-DM-
  HAS). *Role of LMHAs.* Hartford, Connecticut. Power Point
  retrieved from: http://www.ct.gov/dmhas/lib/dmhas/
  presentations/bhrp041410.pdf, 2010.

Evans, O., L. Faulkner, G. Hodo, and D. Mahrer "A quality
  improvement process for state mental health systems" (Rep.
  No. 43(5)). PsycINFO database: Hospital and Community
  Psychiatry, 1992.

Gardner, N. "Modernizing human services: now more than ever"
  (Rep. No. 67(2)). Policy & Practice of Public
  Human Services, 2009.

Guardian Ad Litem Services, Inc. *Guardian Ad Litem Services Satisfaction Survey.* Naugatuck, Connecticut, March 2010.

Guardian Ad Litem Services, Inc. *Guardian Ad Litem Services Administrator's Survey.* Naugatuck, Connecticut, October 2010.

Kind, Viki, MA. *The Caregiver's Path to Compassionate Decision Making:
  Making Choices for Those Who Can't.* Austin: Greenleaf Book
  Group Press, 2010.

Minkoff, K. "Developing standards of care for individuals with
  co-occurring psychiatric and substance use disorders"
  (Rep. No. 52(5)). Psychiatric Services. doi:10.1176/appi.
  ps.52.5.597, 2001.

O'Brien, Aileen et al. "Disengagement from Mental Health Services," Fahemy Division of Mental Health, St. George's University of London. Canmer Terrace, London SW 17 ORE, UK. Singh Health Sciences Research Institute, Warwick Medical School. University of Warwick, Coventry, UK. http://www.academia.edu/427187/Disengagement_From_Mental_Health_Services, 2008.

Patti, Rino, et al. "Seeking better performance through interagency collaboration: prospects and challenges." Southern Area Consortium of Human Services, 2003.

Ring, C. N. "Quality assurance in mental health care: a case study from social work" (Rep. No. 9(6)). Health & Social Care in the Community. doi:10.1046/j.0966-0410.2001.00324.x, Nov 2001.

Savin, H., and S. Kiesling. *Accountable Systems of Behavioral Health Care: A Provider's Guide.* San Francisco: Jossey Bass, 2000.

South Carolina Hospital Association (SCHA). "A Hidden Crisis: South Carolina's Behavioral Health System." https://www.scha.org/files/documents/bh_hiddencrisis_2009.pdf, 2009.

ABOUT THE AUTHOR

An attorney, innovator, and strategist, Michael Mackniak, JD, is the nation's foremost speaker on Interrelated Service Systems. He's also a national certified guardian and a certified brain injury specialist. He focuses on the collaborative development of efficient, effective methods for delivering needed resources to our most at-need populations.

Michael promotes proactive and cooperative planning to avoid costly and ineffective interventions in all service settings. Commissioners, administrators, directors, and clinicians use his practical approach to challenging systems issues in a world of decreasing resources and increasing expectations.

With a law degree from Quinnipiac University, Michael also holds a master's degree in Nonprofit Management from Bay Path University. He provides a team approach to consultation on the most difficult and challenging mental health cases. His programs, implementing The Guardian Model, have received national recognition and multiple awards and honors, including Eli Lily's Welcome Back Award, NAMI's Hero Award, and the 2015 National College of Probate Judge's Isabella Award.

ACKNOWLEDGMENTS

My son Jacob has been an integral part of the writing of this piece. I wish I could be half the man he is at age thirteen.

Thanks to my father who believes it never hurts to try and my mother who questions it all. Special thanks to Kellie, Ryan, and Connor who have always supported my writing. And, of course, to my "lil punkin" Ellie.

Thanks to my partner Sara Valentino who is my rock and the straw that stirs the drink. With me for twenty years, she is the best in our profession and the best friend and partner I could ever ask for. With Angela Caron Hurzeler, Sara has created the program details that make these concepts work. Angela has been the third leg that's vital to our agency's well-balanced stool.

Thanks to Viki Kind who offered needed guidance, support, and cheerleading throughout this project and Dr. Paul T. Amble, MD, who wrote the Foreword.

A very special thanks to Judge James Lawlor and Dr. Ken Marcus who still believe in us.

My sincere thanks also to the following people:

> Our early steering committee of Collette Anderson, Karen Evertson, Gloria Dzerovich, Larry Davidson, and Dr. Paul Amble.

> Simie Whelan, Commissioner Tom Kirk, Commissioner Pat Rehmer, Probate Court Administrator Paul Knierim, and Vincent Russo.

Dr. Ezra Griffith, Sue Graham, Lee Swearingen, and Dr. Charles Dike.

Dr. Matt Snow and Ellen Brotherton.

Judges Fred Anthony, Diane Yamin, Mike Magistralli, Jack Keyes, Bob Killian, and Dan Caruso (and all of their clerks Lori, Pat, Gail, Trish, Tati, Monica, and Kate).

Book editing and production team: Karen Saunders, Patrice Rhodes-Baum, Barbara McNichol, Helena Mariposa, Kelly Johnson, Mark Berardi, Alyvia Kripps, and Kerrie Lian.

ENDNOTES

1   https://www.cms.gov/Research-Statistics-Data-and-Systems/
    Statistics-Trends-and-Reports/NationalHealthExpendData/
    downloads/proj2012.pdf

2   https://www.cms.gov/Research-Statistics-Data-and-Systems/
    Statistics-Trends-and-Reports/NationalHealthExpendData/
    downloads/proj2012.pdf

3   http://www.thenationalcouncil.org/capitol-connector/
    wp-content/blogs.dir/2/files/2014/12/FY2015-omnibus-
    budget-chart.pdf

4   http://www.sentencingproject.org/template/page.cfm?id=107

5   http://www.academia.edu/427187/Disengagement_From_
    Mental_Health_Services

6   O'Brien, Aileen et al, "Disengagement from Mental Health
    Services," (London: http://www.academia.edu/427187/Dis-
    engagement_From_Mental_Health_Services, 2008), 563.

7   Connecticut General Statute

BOOK ORDERING:

Conservative Care, Inc.
www.MichaelMackniak.com
Phone: 203-723-4332
Fax: 203-723-9250

info@michaelmackniak.com

Price: $23.00
(includes shipping
& handling)

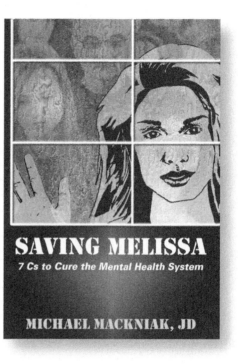

CPSIA information can be obtained at www.ICGtesting.com
Printed in the USA
BVOW08s1827220816

459803BV00001B/10/P

9 780997 421408